Gender and Water, Sanitation and Hygiene

Praise for this book

'A great resource for WASH professionals who want to understand both the basics and the nuances of the link between WASH and gender equality. Because it covers a wide range of WASH sector focus areas – from urban to rural contexts, water resources to sanitation access, gender relations connected to WASH work as well as uniquely female experiences of menstruation, child birth and menopause, it is a worthwhile read for all of us working in or wanting to understand the impacts of WASH on gender.'

Priya Nath, Equality, inclusion and rights advisor, WaterAid

Gender and Water, Sanitation and Hygiene

Edited by
Caroline Sweetman and Louise Medland

Practical ACTION PUBLISHING

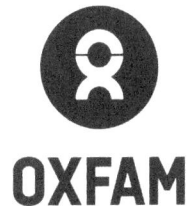

OXFAM

Published by Practical Action Publishing in association with Oxfam GB

Practical Action Publishing Ltd
27a Albert Street, Rugby, Warwickshire, CV21 2SG, UK
www.practicalactionpublishing.org

A catalogue record for this book is available from the British Library.
A catalogue record for this book has been requested from the Library of Congress.

ISBN 978-1-78853-083-5 Paperback
ISBN 978-1-78853-084-2 Hardback
ISBN 978-1-78853-085-9 Epub
ISBN 978-1-78853-086-6 PDF

Citation: Sweetman, C. and Medland, L. (eds) (2019) *Gender and Water, Sanitation and
Hygiene*, Rugby, UK: Practical Action Publishing and Oxford: Oxfam GB. http://dx.doi.
org/10.3362/9781788530866

Since 1974, Practical Action Publishing has published and disseminated books and
information in support of international development work throughout the world.
Practical Action Publishing is a trading name of Practical Action Publishing Ltd
(Company Reg. No. 1159018), the wholly owned publishing company of Practical
Action. Practical Action Publishing trades only in support of its parent charity
objectives and any profits are covenanted back to Practical Action (Charity Reg. No.
247257, Group VAT Registration No. 880 9924 76).

Oxfam is a registered charity in England and Wales (no 202918) and Scotland (SC
039042). Oxfam GB is a member of Oxfam International.

Oxfam GB,
Oxfam House, John Smith Drive,
Oxford, OX4 2JY, UK
www.oxfam.org.uk

Cover photo shows Judith in Kisumu, Kenya, using a new water point at a residential
plot which host several households.
Credit: Patrick Meinhardt, Practical Action photo library, Rugby

Contents

1. Introduction to gender and water, sanitation and hygiene   1
    Louise Medland and Caroline Sweetman

2. No relief: lived experiences of inadequate sanitation
    access of poor urban women in India   17
    Seema Kulkarni, Kathleen O'Reilly & Sneha Bhat

3. Mainstreaming gender in the WASH sector: dilution
    or distillation?   35
    Julie Fisher, Sue Cavill & Brian Reed

4. Mainstreaming gender in WASH: lessons learned from Oxfam's
    experience of Ebola   57
    Simone E. Carter, Luisa Maria Dietrich & Olive Melissa Minor

5. Women's environmental health activism around waste and
    plastic pollution in the coastal wetlands of Yucatán   75
    Anne-Marie Hanson

6. Reframing women's empowerment in water security
    programmes in Western Nepal   91
    Stephanie Leder, Floriane Clement & Emma Karki

7. In troubled waters: water commodification, law, gender,
    and poverty in Bangalore   109
    Kaveri Thara

8. Domesticating water supplies through rainwater
    harvesting in Mumbai   127
    Cat Button

9. Transforming gender relations through water, sanitation,
    and hygiene programming and monitoring in Vietnam   143
    *Caitlin Leahy, Keren Winterford, Tuyen Nghiem, John Kelleher,
    Lee Leong & Juliet Willetts*

10. 'Breaking the silence around menstruation': experiences
    of adolescent girls in an urban setting in India   163
    Shobhita Rajagopal & Kanchan Mathur

11. Resources   179
    Liz Cooke

http://dx.doi.org/10.3362/9781788530866.000

About the editors

Louise Medland is former WASH Resilience Adviser at Oxfam GB. She spent 10 years working in the WASH sector. She now manages a large project aiming to spark a revolution in clean cooking. Email: l.s.medland@lboro.ac.uk

Caroline Sweetman is Editor of the international journal *Gender & Development* and works for Oxfam GB.

Working in Gender and Development

The *Working in Gender and Development series* brings together themed selections of the best articles from the journal *Gender & Development* and other Oxfam publications for development practitioners and policy makers, students, and academics. Titles in the series present the theory and practice of gender-oriented development in a way that records experience, describes good practice, and shares information about resources. Books in the series will contribute to and review current thinking on the gender dimensions of particular development and relief issues.

Other titles in the series are available from www.developmentbookshop. com and include:

Gender-Based Violence
HIV and AIDS
Climate Change and Gender Justice
Gender and the Economic Crisis
Gender, Faith and Development
Gender, Monitoring, Evaluation and Learning
Gender, Business and Enterprise
Gender, Development and Care
Gender and Inequalities
Working with Men for Gender Equality

For further information on the journal please visit www.genderanddevelopment.org

CHAPTER 1

Introduction: Gender and water, sanitation, and hygiene

Caroline Sweetman and Louise Medland

At birth and death, and each day in between, human needs for water, sanitation, and hygiene (WASH) are near-constant. In the most intimate and personal ways, WASH offers 'life-giving or life-threatening potential at some of the most spectacular and mundane moments of life for each of us' (Woodburn, 2016).

The chapters in this collection focus on WASH from the perspective of gender justice and women's rights. WASH is an acronym adopted by the UN in 2007–2008, the International Year of Sanitation. The W of WASH stands for Water, specifically access to safe water for drinking – that is, water free from chemical and biological pollutants. The S stands for Sanitation, specifically access to a toilet (latrine) that safely separates human excreta from humans. The H stands for Hygiene, specifically focusing on public health and the transmission of faecal-oral diseases. WASH replaced earlier approaches, in the early decades of development, which began by focusing on water provision, followed by the addition of sanitation, referred to as WATSAN. The move to the language of WASH signals a wider agenda, recognizing the need for a range of complementary political, economic, and socio-cultural changes and measures needed in addition to services and infrastructure, to realize the ultimate goal of WASH: human health, wellbeing, and development.

While WASH is intensely personal, as suggested above, it is also about power, inequality, development, and social justice. On the eve of World Water Day in 2013, more people possessed a mobile phone than a toilet (see UN News, 2013). Global access to WASH has improved, in particular during the era of the Millennium Development Goals (MDGs). From 1990 to 2010, mortality from diarrhoeal diseases fell by 41.9 per cent, from 2.5 million to 1.4 million (Lozano et al., 2012). However, this story masks another, of lack of progress in particular regions. Unimproved sanitation and unimproved water remain among the top 12 risk factors in most of sub-Saharan Africa, where diarrhoea remains a leading cause of death (Liu et al., 2012). In 2015, as the MDGs gave way to the new era of the Sustainable Development Goals (SDGs), 663 million people – 1 in 10 – still lacked access to safe water, while 2.4 billion people lacked improved sanitation facilities (UNICEF/WHO, 2015: 4).

http://dx.doi.org/10.3362/9781788530866.001

Social taboos around excretion and body waste exist the world over, and embarrassment – even disgust – discourages discussions that highlight the urgency and injustice of the issues. The people who lack water and sanitation usually live and die away from the gaze of the powerful. If they become ill, or die, due to unmet WASH needs, this can go relatively unnoticed by those of us fortunate enough to be able to drink and wash in clean water supplies and relieve ourselves using modern toilets. Safe sanitation channels our waste away from us before we even have to see it, let alone work out how to dispose of it without exposing ourselves or others to the risk of infection, embarrassment, or violence due to stigma.

Writers in this collection offer perspectives on WASH from the point of gender justice and women's rights. They highlight the importance of WASH provision for women and girls, in their own right and as carers for families and communities. WASH is a human right, and a key to women's empowerment. In the next section of this Introduction, we examine the gender aspects of WASH in more detail, before moving on to consider current policy and programme approaches to WASH that aim to address women's and girls' needs and interests.

WASH: a gender analysis

Women and girls experience sanitation needs differently from men. The powerful taboos and stigmas connected to defecation or urination mentioned above are common in human societies, and create secrecy, shame, and disgust around excretion. These obviously affect everyone. However, women's bodily functions are commonly associated in patriarchal societies with a requirement for privacy and the notion that body functions should be kept secret. Women who do not manage to achieve this are often punished, sometimes with violence. The two sets of ideas and beliefs about excretion and female bodies intersect to create particularly acute problems for women in households and communities without water and sanitation. While men may be able to relieve themselves with relative ease and will not face major reprisals if they are seen doing so, the picture is very different for women.

In their chapter in this collection, Seema Kulkarni, Kathleen O'Reilly, and Sneha Bhat give a vivid account of the sanitation-related violence and harassment of women in slum areas of two Indian cities, Pune and Jaipur. This chapter paints a vivid picture of women's and girls' daily struggle of finding somewhere to defecate in Indian slums and highlights that even where toilets are present, the high numbers of users and lack of cleaning leave them unusable. For women, the experience of open defecation is made worse by the harassment and abuse they endure from men and boys.

Menstruation, pregnancy, childbirth and its aftermath, and female menopause all create needs for water and sanitation that are specific to women, and these specifically female bodily functions create hygiene, health, and well-being problems that can affect women and girls in a range of ways. In their chapter in the collection, Shobhita Rajagopal and Kanchan Mathur focus on the experiences of adolescent girls in Jaipur, Rajasthan. As they state:

> The onset of menstruation, and the practices associated with it, are areas shrouded in silence across many cultures in South Asia; yet they bring many challenges. On the one hand, puberty is a period of rapid transition for adolescent girls, and a critical time for identity formation; on the other, prevailing patriarchal ideologies, cultural taboos and traditional practices exclude women and girls from various activities including school attendance, reinforcing gender inequalities (Shobhita Rajagopal and Kanchan Mathur, p. 163).

Menstruation is commonly associated with pollution, and many societies worldwide see it as a reason for excluding and segregating women from family and community life for a week or more, each month. Some women are expected in some communities to remain within their homes, or in a special room, and there are taboos on handling and preparing food. Rituals may be required to purify them afterwards. The cloths used during menstruation need to be concealed from men and boys and often also from other women and girls, and washed in secret.

Unmet WASH needs add to the dangers of childbearing for women in poverty in the global South. A recent World Health Organization (WHO) study reviewed data on the estimated 287,000 maternal deaths that occurred between 2003 and 2009 – most of which were avoidable (Say et al., 2014: 323). Globally, 10.7 per cent of maternal deaths were related to sepsis (infections that can be cut dramatically by hand-washing on the part of midwives and health staff). These sepsis-related maternal deaths were almost all in developing countries, and the proportion of such deaths was highest in southern Asia, at 13.7 per cent (ibid.: 328). The study highlighted the importance of focusing beyond the technical aspects of WASH – the provision of water and sanitation services and infrastructure – to the social factors (including attitudinal change and health education) needed to deliver WASH for all.

In addition to experiencing their own personal needs for WASH, women shoulder responsibility for the WASH needs of others. The gender division of labour in most societies worldwide puts women in charge of ensuring family wellbeing, health, and hygiene. The burden that accompanies this responsibility is immensely heavier in households and communities without clean, safe, accessible, and affordable water and toilets. For women in poverty, the modern machines that have lightened the work of laundry are unaffordable. Yet the modern economy is centred on the idea of a paid worker who is available to do their job for 8 or 10 hours a day – or more. Unpaid care work presents a practical barrier to all such dreams. In 2014, the immense workload associated with unpaid care – including WASH – was highlighted as a human rights violation by the UN Special Rapporteur on Extreme Poverty, because:

> The unequal distribution, intensity, and lack of recognition and support of unpaid care work undermines the dignity and autonomy of women caregivers and obstructs the enjoyment of several human rights – including economic, social, cultural and political rights – on an equal basis with men (Sepúlveda Carmona and Donald, 2014: 444).

A recent study of 24 sub-Saharan African countries estimated that 13.54 million adult women (and 3.36 million children) spend more than 30 minutes each day collecting water for their households (Graham et al., 2016: 2). Lack of sanitation for an entire household places the onus on women as carers to protect their children from the insecurity of open defecation – in particular, daughters; the women in Seema Kulkarni et al.'s study, mentioned above, stated that they feared for their daughters' safety more than their own, and accompanied them when they needed to visit open defecation sites.

WASH also affects women carers when family members fall ill from avoidable waterborne diseases. The figures given at the start of this chapter speak for themselves about the workload and emotional anguish felt by women caring for family members suffering from waterborne diseases. In their chapter in this collection, Simone E. Carter, Luisa Maria Dietrich, and Olive Melissa Minor focus on the lessons to be learned from Oxfam's Ebola response. The social and cultural dynamics driving the Ebola outbreak concerned women's role in caring for the ill, the dying, and the deceased, including the social expectation that women perform the rituals of preparing bodies for burial:

> The research showed that the social expectation that families would care for their loved ones during life and observe cultural practices of care for bodies after death created undeniable risks for those involved in overseeing and delivering care, particularly for women. A 'good' mother or wife was seen as one who cared for and provided for the sick, however in Ebola she was explicitly told not to provide care and, in fact, told that providing care for the sick and deceased increased risk to the outbreak and its spread. This was because they are more likely to come into contact with bodily fluids or blood which is the primary method of transmission (Simone Carter, Luisa Maria Dietrich, and Olive Melissa Minor, p. 63).

The time spent by women carers shoring up family wellbeing and health in the face of unmet WASH needs could be used in many ways. It prevents education, earning income, taking part in politics, or sleep. Leisure is often non-existent. In addition to the time that reducing the drudgery associated with WASH would save, it would benefit women's physical and psychological health. WASH labour is heavy labour. In a study of six communities in South Africa, women and children carried water weighing an average of 19.5 kg over an average distance of 335 m. Sixty-nine per cent reported spinal pain, with the potential to lead to muscular-skeletal disorders (Geere et al., 2010: 1).

This analysis shows that unmet WASH needs affecting women's daily lives also perpetuate gender inequality and women's subordination. Down the decades, the WASH sector has engaged with these issues in a range of different ways.

WASH programming to support women's rights and gender justice

In their chapter in this collection, Julie Fisher, Sue Cavill, and Brian Reed take a historical look at the evolution of the WASH approach to women and gender from the vantage point of the papers submitted over the years to the Water, Engineering and Development Centre International Conference, now in its 40th year. They offer a fascinating account of how the WASH sector has been influenced by the parallel development of the fields of Women in Development (WID) and, later, Gender and Development (GAD).

Julie Fisher et al. point out particular milestones in the journey to achieve water and sanitation for all. These include the 1977 United Nations Water Conference at Mar del Plata, the 1981–1990 International Drinking Water and Sanitation Decade, and the International Conference on Water and the Environment in Dublin, held in January 1992.

The Dublin Conference paid direct and explicit attention to women's key and central role in providing, maintaining, managing, and protecting water. Agenda 21, which came out of the Rio Conference on Environment and Development, recognized the role of women in water management (see the Rio Declaration, Chapter 18). The International Decade for Action, 'Water for Life' (2005–2015), called for women's participation and involvement in water-related development efforts.

The start of the Sustainable Development Goals (SDGs) has marked an intensified focus on water, sanitation, and hygiene: by 2030, Goal 6 aims to 'ensure availability and sustainable management of water and sanitation for all'. Target 1 is 'universal and equitable access to safe and affordable drinking water', and Target 2 is 'access to adequate and equitable sanitation and hygiene for all and end open defecation, paying special attention to the needs of women and girls and those in vulnerable situations'.[1]

The SDG challenge to 'leave no one behind' has been taken up in the WASH sector, through its commitment to universal provision of water. But to do this by the deadline of 2030 would be a gargantuan task even if SDG 6 had fewer limitations.[2] The SDGs have built on and developed an awareness of the links between complex inequalities and poverty. Leaving no one behind in WASH – and responding to the related current 'equity and inclusion' agenda (discussed by Julie Fisher et al. in their chapter) – means involving women in planning and programming. It means adopting a rights-based approach – including women's rights and gender justice as key intersecting components (Gosling, 2010).

Parallel to these milestones in WASH policymaking, WASH practitioners in development and humanitarian organizations have also found their work shaped by the impetus to integrate gender issues into their work in response to calls from women's movements since the 1970s. Julie Fisher et al. trace how WID and GAD approaches have been taken on in the WASH sector.

Since the early days, awareness of needing to design infrastructure and technology to meet the needs of women has grown in the sector. Often, this has focused on security, in response to the realities of the harassment and violence women and girls can face when using WASH facilities. Programmes have involved women in planning, implementation, and running of WASH facilities, in both development and humanitarian sectors, in villages, peri-urban slums, and camps for displaced people. The underlying rationales vary. Some programmes focus on efficiency and meeting the needs of children, families, or communities, drawing on women's knowledge, skills, and energies but not challenging or seeking to change existing unequal gender roles or workloads.

But as understandings of the link between power and economic poverty have strengthened, programming has grappled with the question of how WASH provision links to women's empowerment and gender equality. Today, as Julie Fisher et al. remind us, women's empowerment has become widely accepted as a legitimate and important goal in WASH programming. Involving women at all levels of programming is seen by many local, national, and international NGOs as important not only because it makes it more likely that projects will be useful and sustainable, but also because this potentially shifts attitudes to women leaders in their families and communities.

Chapters in this collection focus on a range of topics and demonstrate how development and humanitarian WASH programming has addressed gender equality and women's rights.

Women's voices on the right to water: governance and accountability

Women living in poverty remain distanced from any power to influence – let alone decide – water policies. Issues of governance and accountability are critical if policies and practices are ever to reflect the realities of the poorest women.

Kaveri Thara's chapter provides a case study of a context where the notion of the right to water has been contested for nearly three decades, and where women living in extreme poverty are asserting that it should be the state, not private households, who should pay. This study of resistance to cost-recovery strategies in water provision in Bangalore demonstrates that the poorest people are actually forced to pay more for water than the better-off. Women are marginalized from policymaking.

Kaveri Thara's chapter focuses on Bangalore where (as in other cities in the global South and North) decision-making on water provision remains largely top-down, and involves technical experts and specialists. There is little involvement of the poorest women and men who are most affected by state decision-making as they are least capable of turning to the market to meet water supply and sanitation needs. Women and men living in poverty have few means beyond protest to articulate their views. After protests failed to stop the city moving to cost recovery, women have retained their vision of universal WASH, which rests on free access and notions of social justice:

> Women continue to see water – and claim it – as a public good, something they have a right to, by virtue of having life, and by virtue of their poverty. This response needs to be contextualized within a long history of water provision that acknowledged their human right to water, by providing the poor with public taps (Kaveri Thara, p. 199).

One strategy to subvert the system adopted by women in Kaveri Thara's study is to use social relationships with local government officials, who hope for continued political support in return for negotiating for access for free water from public taps that are now locked.

In contrast, several chapters in this collection focus on the ways NGOs have involved women in the planning and governance of WASH interventions that have a conscious focus on reaching the poor. In locations where NGOs have taken on the role of WASH provider, they have typically involved communities in infrastructure and service provision, often using participatory planning methods. As Julie Fisher et al. mention in their chapter in this collection, gender analysis tools and frameworks – many of them for emergency programming including WASH – evolved through the 1980s to 1990s, as gender mainstreaming in development gathered pace. The tools and frameworks aimed to provide details of gender roles and relations in communities, and to involve women in the design, implementation, and evaluation of WASH programming.

Also in this collection, Caitlin Leahy, Keren Winterford, Tuyen Nghiem, John Kelleher, Lee Leong, and Juliet Willetts present the results of empirical research conducted in central Vietnam in 2016 into WASH initiatives. In particular, the authors were interested in assessing the impact of a Gender and WASH Monitoring Tool (GWMT), developed by Plan International Australia and Plan Vietnam. In this chapter, they provide an example of how this tool was used to shed light on changes reported by women and men of different ages and ethnicities who were affected by WASH projects, and consider the reasons for the changes. Their chapter – and the tool they discuss – draws on a range of gender-analysis concepts, and uncovers changes in gender relations and power dynamics at both household and community levels. This helps explore the extent to which both the practical interests of women and the goal of gender equality can be influenced and changed by WASH policies and programming.

Simone E. Carter et al.'s chapter also offers insights into gender, governance, and accountability in the fragile context of the Ebola response in West Africa. They show how careful and detailed research involving women is essential to ensure effective and empowering responses to WASH needs in humanitarian crisis. However, their case study shows how an emergency response in a fragile context where government is struggling can become top-down and less participatory at the precise moment that local knowledge and buy-in becomes critical. In the Ebola national response, a male-dominated and militarized response prevented women's voices from being heard.

Empowering women through WASH: understanding what this means

By 2017, many WASH programmes had a gender equality or women's empowerment aim. Yet understanding of what empowerment looks like, how to support women to become empowered, and what the scope is for WASH to promote this, remains patchy. In many development organizations, there is an expectation that knowing how to work on 'gender' or 'women' is widely understood. However, the ways WASH can achieve this deserves more open discussion than it sometimes receives in organizations where gender mainstreaming is now a requirement. In the process of commissioning and editing this collection (initially articles for the journal *Gender & Development*) the notion of empowerment was used in many different ways in discussions between the editors and authors. It seems that WASH practitioners can commonly feel that they are expected to take women's empowerment as a given, and know how to do it (personal communications, May 2017).

Understandings of what women's empowerment is, who defines it, and how it is supported by development and humanitarian actors have been many and varied. In their overview of gender mainstreaming in the WASH sector Julie Fisher et al. trace a concern for the sustainability of water and sanitation programming, and the role of women in ensuring this. This concern has been accompanied by a commitment to ease women's workloads, increase their ability to produce and earn money as a result of water provision, and ultimately to empower women through WASH. The idea that a WASH programme can contribute to change in gender relations in wider society is also commonly mooted by gender specialists working alongside WASH practitioners. But how can this happen?

As the chapters in this collection show, examining WASH from a gender perspective involves extending the gaze beyond the important technical concerns of services and infrastructure to focus on social relations: in particular, thinking about power. Without the power to secure essential resources including access to water, sanitation, and the ability to practise good hygiene, both personal and domestic, human agency is constrained and there can be little meaningful human achievement. Women and men without power to obtain water and sanitation are trapped in a vicious circle in which it is hard to see how they can move forward in any substantive way. WASH is thus intrinsically empowering. The challenge is to ensure all can gain access to it; that no one – and in particular, no woman – is left behind.

However, the language of empowerment has become ubiquitous, and in many cases means little. Gender and development's understanding of women's empowerment originally arose from global women's movements in the 1980s and 1990s, and was founded on a vision of Southern women's right to define the concept for themselves (Moser, 1993). In this original vision, there was a clear – and limited – role for development organizations. While they could offer financial support, technical input, and other support as required and requested by women in the global South, development organizations were not free to impose an outsider agenda and activities.

Yet programmes with an empowerment aim often do impose on women at the grassroots. SDG 6 has a target on protecting and restoring water ecosystems, and Anne-Marie Hanson's chapter on this topic focuses on women's environmental activism around waste and plastic pollution. She highlights that while women's participation and the 'needs of women' can be a central component of project or programme design, the power dynamics are often not empowering. There is little evidence that such programmes actually benefit women, or allow them to do more than just 'participate' by being 'recipients of an intervention'. Too often, we use the language of empowerment, but still expect women to take on passive roles.

Empowerment and WASH in the era of 'leave no one behind': Gender 2.0

Currently, the UN's 'leave no one behind' approach, with its emphasis on the link between complex inequalities and marginalization, is creating real impetus for development practitioners to focus freshly on power and empowerment (Mangubhai and Capraro, 2015). A host of inequalities (e.g. race, caste, disability) encourage an analysis of how people are marginalized for many different reasons. But 'leave no one behind' does not mean a departure from the global commitment to gender equality and women's empowerment.[3] Instead, it means a shift to what could be called 'Gender 2.0': the empowerment of all women and girls, including those marginalized by other aspects of identity, for example caste, race, or being lone heads of household.

For WASH practitioners focusing on gender inequality and women's empowerment, this means working with women in a community to find out who is most marginalized, why, and a commitment to working with women to design and implement WASH programmes that benefit everyone. In their chapter, Stephanie Leder, Floriane Clement, and Emma Karki provide a case study which shows the importance of doing this. They focus on research findings from four villages in western Nepal, where two internationally funded WASH programmes specifically aimed to empower women, by improving access to water for both domestic and productive uses.

As the chapter shows, the programmes had the ambitious aspiration of transforming women into rural entrepreneurs and grassroots leaders. However, impact assessment showed how the work had benefited some women more than others. Differences in identity and power relations between women – depending on issues including age, marital status, caste, and household prosperity – led to some women being able to take advantage of the WASH programmes more than others. There is a clear message that water programmes must recognize and address difference between women if the poorest and most disadvantaged women are to benefit. While these insights are not new, the focus on 'leave no one behind' challenges WASH practitioners to design programmes designed to empower the most marginalized.

Caitlin Leahy et al.'s chapter, mentioned above, offers evidence of how age and ethnicity alter individuals' experience of a particular intervention aimed to support everyone equally. This reminds us of the limitations of focusing on a single category of 'women', and/or a focus only on gender inequality. Projects need to focus on difference among women, and ensure that the more marginalized among them are able to secure the fullest benefits of WASH.

Universal WASH access: the challenge of financing

Achieving universal WASH coverage involves challenging the complex economic, social, and political inequalities that constrain the poorest people from accessing WASH, ensuring that WASH is affordable for all. It will also involve devising ways of financing WASH which ensure it can reach the poorest women and men, ensuring that the universal right to water is realized. This will require the costs of providing WASH to be correctly calculated and covered, including operation and maintenance of systems and administration; finding capital at affordable rates to invest in infrastructure suitable to reach the hardest to find people living in rural isolation and urban sprawl; and finding the knowledge, expert skills, and input to invest in the sector.

As the challenges of financing WASH are addressed, poor women are rarely if ever included in these discussions. Solutions tend to worsen their situation as primary collectors and users of water. In her chapter, Kaveri Thara focuses on women living in poverty in an urban area of Bangalore, tracing their struggles to obtain water in the face of evolving policies on water provision. Despite recognition of the right to water, the issue of cost and affordability is critical here as elsewhere. The poorest, both rural and urban, are often adversely affected by failures in infrastructure provision and are less able to access the services provided by infrastructures when they are available, with affordability highlighted as the key determinant to access (Estache and Fay, 2007; Briceno-Garmendia et al., 2004).

As Kaveri Thara's chapter shows, in contexts with strong histories of rights-based development and liberation, women at the grassroots are resisting the monetization of water in principle, while in practice their need for it requires them to scrape together the money to buy it. While the advantages of the technologies that accompany this process are emphasized by the authorities – piped water is seen as saving time and increasing mobility, as well as delivering a higher-quality resource – women retort that the requirement to pay for water outweighs the benefits. City authorities need to be accountable to all, including women in poverty.

A complementary chapter in this collection comes from Cat Button, who examines a solution to water shortages in urban Mumbai that focuses on a technology to be purchased by the better-off city residents. This is rainwater harvesting, undertaken at the level of individual households. As the chapter points out, this solution to water shortages shifts responsibility for water provision from city authorities to private households. While it can be 'sold' as giving residents more control, and could also change the gendered power balance of water provision by ending the need for women to collect water, these benefits need to be balanced against the fact that poor households are not able to adopt rainwater harvesting. As Cat Button points out, power, gender inequality, and environmental justice are central to WASH provision.

Learning what works in WASH programming

Learning from programmes still continues to be a challenge in many development and humanitarian organizations, requiring significant investment of resources to do properly, and a receptivity to reflecting critically on the challenges of programmes. The chapter by Simone E. Carter, Luisa Maria Dietrich, and Olive Melissa Minor in this collection focuses on Oxfam's learning from its work in the Ebola crisis of 2014–2015. This case study highlights a range of issues which staff involved in Oxfam's response considered the most important to learn from for future interventions. The first issue was the militarized nature of this large-scale response to Ebola, in countries where health and other systems were struggling. Second, there was limited participation of women and other traditionally marginalized groups in the planning and implementation of the response. Third, the impact of a narrow gender mainstreaming lens on programme effectiveness led to a focus on women and unpaid care work at the expense of a wider approach incorporating the roles of men and boys. In Oxfam, a sound gender analysis was provided by a team of professionals from a range of technical and social development backgrounds. This analysis provided a foundation for an appropriate and effective response.

The chapter by Carter et al. also highlights the importance of comprehensive gender equality standards in WASH humanitarian response, but argues that even these cannot deliver the best possible programming. To do this, emergency responses are needed that are informed by a robust body of gender mainstreaming guidelines. These can address gender issues arising in specific contexts, and enhance women's participation in WASH emergency programming.

This chapter is a case study of one particular organization's specific work in contribution to the wider Ebola response; but stepping back to widen the focus to the whole response (involving UN agencies, governments, and international NGOs) is also important, to give a picture of progress on gender mainstreaming at scale. A key issue highlighted by gender specialists working in emergencies relates to the current humanitarian coordination system (where 'clusters' of organizations have specific lead roles in coordinating a response). There is a WASH cluster (led by UNICEF), but there is no specific cluster leading on gender, and awareness of and appreciation of the importance of gender mainstreaming is left to the individual organizations within the clusters.

Breaking the silence and working on social norms

As a sector, WASH is evolving a growing understanding of the importance of the social and cultural contexts in which people use water and sanitation. The 'H' of Hygiene in the WASH acronym reminds us that WASH is as much about health education and working to challenge social norms that harm health and hygiene as it is about services and infrastructure.

Simone Carter et al.'s chapter on Oxfam's Ebola response provides an extreme example of the sensitivities that can exist around social norm change. As stated earlier, WASH may be connected to rituals of life and death. The women wishing to bathe the bodies of their loved ones had to choose between obeying a health message asking them not to, or risk continuing spreading Ebola by ignoring this message. It is very sensitive to question – let alone challenge – people's ideas and beliefs rooted in duty, affection, and loss.

Since the start of this current decade, the WASH sector has developed its work around women's gender-specific WASH needs that arise from discriminatory and stigmatizing social norms around female bodies. As highlighted above, gender-specific WASH issues remain extremely hard to voice even to female relatives or schoolteachers, let alone to male relatives, or men outside the family. Yet the details of how women and girls negotiate through these challenges each day and month of their lives, and how their requirements for WASH change over their lifecycles and prevent or enable them to participate in activities outside the home – critically, in formal education or in paid employment or income-earning – need to be a critical part of WASH planning and provision. This information needs to be known to policymakers in the institutions that provide WASH services and infrastructure.

In their chapter, Shobhita Rajagopal and Kanchan Mathur discuss a state-sponsored intervention to promote menstrual hygiene through the provision of sanitary pads to schoolgirls. Their discussion reveals the inadequacy of this response in a context of gender inequality, stigma around menstruation and women's bodies, and poverty. While the provision of 'modern' sanitary protection may be welcomed by many, the affordability of modern technologies is an issue, as is the need for health and relationships education, and work with both young women and young men to challenge the gender inequality that lies behind attitudes to women, women's bodies, and sex. A narrow focus on 'menstrual hygiene' is not sufficient to ensure girls' experience of the onset of menstruation is positive, nor to fully address the issue of girls being able to move around outside their homes (attending schools or indeed earning income).

A final point on social norms concerns the need for professional knowledge from many different fields, to ensure the 'H' in Hygiene is delivered. Focusing on social norm change relating to women's care load, including water collection and sanitation, is obviously something that can be done as part of a WASH sector response, but may draw on the expertise of colleagues from different backgrounds, as in Oxfam's Ebola response. WASH is a complex field which needs to bring together the combined expertise of grassroots women and men, with the engineers, architects, city planners, and other professionals tasked with delivering WASH services and infrastructure. WASH also requires other disciplines, including community development workers involved in health education, sociologists, and gender specialists. This can ensure a holistic programme that addresses social norms alongside technical water and sanitation infrastructure and service provision. Challenging the notion that unpaid care is women's work and suggesting that men can also do it is an important element of all programming aiming to support women's empowerment.

Partnership with women's organizations in their WASH-related action

The personal and daily connection between women and the natural environment created by the constant struggle to obtain water and ensure good health and hygiene for families has led many women to become custodians of natural resources. Household and residential garbage management is largely seen as an issue of cleanliness and health, linked to women's domestic responsibilities.

In her chapter in this collection, Anne-Marie Hanson focuses on these issues in the context of an exploration of women's environmental activism around waste and plastic pollution, in coastal Yucatán, Mexico. In these small coastal communities in Mexico women have assumed many of the responsibilities for improving urban conditions and preventing waterborne diseases through community-based organized waste management and education activities.

This activism is centred on sustaining everyday lives in the absence of formal policymaking to protect natural resources and meet needs for rubbish collection, water provision, and sanitation. Anne-Marie Hanson shows how this activism is often invisible to planners who focus on large-scale technical development programming, in which women are seen as passive beneficiaries. Women in poverty are even less likely than men to have a significant say in the decisions about the positioning and design of homes, settlements, and infrastructure.

As we have seen, in the WASH sector, the struggle to provide WASH infrastructure and services is leading to partnerships between the state, NGOs, and private sector institutions. However, the idea of partnerships with social justice movements – including women's movements – is an innovative and promising idea that offers the promise of real change. Rights-based development based on equity and inclusion requires inviting women's organizations into WASH policymaking and planning spaces. In Anne-Marie Hanson's chapter, in the small towns all along the coast of Yucatán, women are the main advocates for community waste management, forming grassroots recycling and composting groups, as well as inter-municipal garbage alliances.

Conclusion

The chapters in this collection aim to offer a range of interesting and thought-provoking views on key challenges to achieving universal access to WASH by 2030. The chapters give examples of the many ways in which the WASH sector has grappled with the challenge of integrating gender equality and women's rights into this most critical of development and humanitarian sectors. Over the past four decades there has been increasing acknowledgement that it is social and political marginalization and complex inequalities – including gender inequality – that drive apparently economic and technical deprivations. This has not only created a different and more accurate analysis of the causes of the problems, but also suggests a set of strategies which are more likely to bring about sustainable solutions, if the political will is there to implement them.

About the contributors

Caroline Sweetman is Editor of *Gender & Development*.

Louise Medland is former WASH Resilience Adviser at Oxfam GB. She spent 10 years working in the WASH sector. She now manages a large project aiming to spark a revolution in clean cooking. Email: l.s.medland@lboro.ac.uk

Notes

1. For further and more detailed information on Goal 6 and its targets, see http://www.un.org/sustainabledevelopment/water-and-sanitation [accessed 29 June 2017].
2. SDG 6 lacks a headline focus on hygiene, and has targets on water and sanitation only. The SDG indicators remain focused on the technology of service provision rather than the wider and more complex considerations required to deliver water, sanitation, and hygiene for all.
3. For a full gender analysis of 'leave no one behind', see Stuart and Woodroffe (2016).

References

Briceno-Garmendia, C., Estache, A., and Shafik, N. (2004) *Infrastructure Services in Developing Countries: Access, Quality, Costs and Policy Reform*, World Bank Policy Research Working Paper 3468, Washington, DC: World Bank.

Estache, A. and Fay, M. (2007) *Current Debates on Infrastructure Policy*, Policy Research Working Paper 4410, Washington, DC: World Bank, Poverty Reduction and Economic Management Vice-Presidency.

Geere, J.-A.L., Hunter, P.R., and Jagals, P. (2010) 'Domestic water carrying and its implications for health: a review and mixed methods pilot study in Limpopo Province, South Africa', *Environmental Health* 9: 52.

Gosling, L. (2010) *Equity and Inclusion: A Rights-Based Approach*, London: WaterAid.

Graham, J.P., Hirai, M., and Kim, S.-S. (2016) 'An analysis of water collection labor among women and children in 24 sub-Saharan African countries', *PLoS ONE* 11(6): e0155981.

Liu, L., Johnson, H.L., Cousens, S., Perin, J., Scott, S., Lawn, J.E., Rudan, I., Campbell, H., Cibulskis, R., Li, M., Mathers, C., and Black, R.E. (2012) 'Global, regional and national causes of child mortality: an updated systematic analysis for 2010 with time trends since 2000', *The Lancet* 379(9832): 2151–61.

Lozano, R., et al. (2012) 'Global and regional mortality from 235 causes of death for 20 age groups in 1990 and 2010: a systematic analysis for the Global Burden of Disease Study 2010', *The Lancet* 380 (9859): 2095–128.

Mangubhai, J.P. and Capraro, C. (2015) '"Leave no one behind" and the challenge of intersectionality: Christian Aid's experience of working with single and Dalit women in India', *Gender & Development* 23(2): 261–77.

Moser, C. (1993) *Gender Planning and Development: Theory, Practice and Training*, London and New York: Routledge.

Say, L., Chou, D., Gemmill, A., Tunçalp, O., Moller, A.-B., Daniels, J., Gülmezoglu, A.M., Temmerman, M., and Alkema, L. (2014) 'Global causes of maternal death: a WHO systematic analysis', *The Lancet* 2(6): e323–33.

Sepúlveda Carmona, M. and Donald, K. (2014) 'What does care have to do with human rights? Analysing the impact on women's rights and gender equality', *Gender & Development* 22(3): 441–57.

Stuart, E. and Woodroffe, J. (2016) 'Leaving no-one behind: can the Sustainable Development Goals succeed where the Millennium Development Goals lacked?' *Gender & Development* 24(1): 69–81.

UNICEF/World Health Organization (WHO) (2015) *Progress on Sanitation and Drinking Water: 2015 Update and MDG Assessment* [pdf], Geneva: WHO <https://www.wssinfo.org/fileadmin/user_upload/resources/JMP-Update-report-2015_English.pdf> [accessed 29 June 2017].

UN News (2013) 'Deputy UN chief calls for urgent action to tackle global sanitation crisis', UN News, 21 March [online] <http://www.un.org/apps/news/story.asp?NewsID=44452#.WVD2eevyvct> [accessed 29 June 2017].

Woodburn, H. (2016) 'Where do we go from here? WASH in the SDGs' [blog], *Huffington Post*, 1 June <http://www.huffingtonpost.com/hanna-woodburn/where-do-we-go-from-here-_2_b_7490146.html> [accessed 29 June 2017].

CHAPTER 2

No relief: lived experiences of inadequate sanitation access of poor urban women in India

Seema Kulkarni, Kathleen O'Reilly and Sneha Bhat

Abstract

The provision of sanitation in India has attracted much attention, but research and policies focusing on gender in relation to sanitation often fail to focus on sanitation-related violence against women (VAW). This chapter focuses on research in Pune (in Maharashtra) and Jaipur (in Rajasthan). It offers evidence of slum-dwelling women's experiences of harassment and violence related to poor or absent sanitation facilities. In addition, it explores the strategies that women adopt to minimise risk and stress. Sanitation-related violence shows the connections between slum geographies and unequal intra-slum relationships of gender, caste, and economic and marital status, and the types of sanitation facilities available. These different identities shape women's experiences of VAW and they commonly blame men from 'outside' or 'other' groups, affecting their ability to act as a united group against violence. While sanitation is inadequate and inappropriate for women's needs across castes, community cohesion and the chances of collective action and advocacy to address sanitation needs are also compromised by tensions between groups in the slum.

Keywords: Gender; psychosocial stress; sanitation; urban; violence

Introduction

The need for urban sanitation in India is clear. In this chapter, we seek to unravel the relationship between violence against women (VAW) and sanitation, focusing on its details, specifics, and its impact at different levels, on individuals and society. By analysing the stories of slum-dwelling women, we aim to offer insights into what the absence of sanitation means for women and girls living in poverty in urban India. What emerges is an understanding of both their individual struggles and the unequal relationships that hold India's gendered urban sanitation crisis in place, affecting the ability of some slum communities to take collective action to lobby for solutions.

The chapter is based on research undertaken between October 2013 and May 2014, in Pune (Maharashtra) and Jaipur (Rajasthan). It involved a number

http://dx.doi.org/10.3362/9781788530866.002

of local non-government organisations (NGOs).[1] The research was undertaken to capture urban poor women's experiences and vulnerabilities due to inadequate sanitation. Our findings offer detailed evidence drawn from observation of real life, on poor urban women's experiences of violence and harassment related to inadequate provision and maintenance of public and community toilets (PTs), and women's continuing use of open defecation (OD) sites as a last resort. The chapter reveals some of the multitude of coping mechanisms that women have adopted to minimise risk and psychosocial stresses. These tend to operate at the level of the individual and her household. Collective action is shaped by the strong sense of identity with caste/ethnic/religious groups in the slum, which affects women's experience of VAW itself, as well as their analysis of the roots of the problems they face.

Our primary question as we began our research was, 'If VAW is symptomatic of power inequalities in society, then how do those inequalities manifest themselves in women's psychosocial stress and translate into women's decisions about where to relieve themselves?' Our findings were striking since they show women experiencing sanitation-related psychological stress happening within a context of complex inequalities including gender, class, caste/ethnic/religious, and economic inequalities, which together create social and political disadvantages, 'precarious livelihoods, unemployment, environmental pollution, and more' (McFarlane *et al.* 2014, 9). Intra-household relations, and intra-slum relationships of gender, caste, and marital status, matter deeply for women, and affect their experience of VAW related to inadequate sanitation (Doron and Jeffrey 2014). Simply put, multiple inequalities and slum geographies mattered most for women's experiences of psychosocial stress.

Gendered struggles for safe sanitation spaces

A body of research and policy on gender and sanitation links lack of adequate sanitation in urban slums to insecurity of land tenure, due to the threat of resettlement (McFarlane *et al.* 2014), uncertain access to water (Hirve *et al.* 2015), and poverty/affordability (Kwiringira *et al.* 2014). Constraints on women's access to PTs – commonly seen as the answer in communities where people lack individual household latrines (IHLs) – include physical ability/mobility, distance, route location and condition, facility design, and an insufficient number of toilet stalls. Solutions to lack of sanitation include advocacy for obtaining and maintaining PTs, making IHLs more affordable, and efforts to promote community cohesion and greater links between people to lessen sanitation-related risks. These solutions include both technical and social elements.

Urban sanitation policy based on technical solutions alone will not result in access to modern sanitation for all. In addition to technical and infrastructural issues, unequal social relations – including gender inequality, intersecting with other inequalities including religion and caste – create discrimination and inequality leading to different experiences of sanitation. Some literature on gender and sanitation recognises identity-based discrimination against women of particular religion or caste, unaffordable cost, and bans on particular women using facilities due to personal whim of the attendant (Actionaid 2013; Osumanu and Kosoe 2013).

PTs, while seen as the best option to manage slum sanitation (Scouten and Mathenge 2010), present gendered hazards for women and children, unless they are well-planned. Toilet blocks are often unlit, making them attractive for illegal activities (e.g. drug use), and for human predators who wait, knowing women or children will come and use them. While women and their families want sanitation facilities, they are therefore wary of using shared or public sanitation facilities that may put them at risk. Maintenance of PTs is commonly a problem due to resources and to lack of buy-in from stakeholders including users.

As a result, PTs often go unused because no one takes responsibility for them (Bapat and Agarwal 2003). If they are insecure or dangerous, filthy, without water, broken, too costly, or closed at night, women will take the risk of going to urinate and defecate in the open air, in locations referred to by WASH professionals and urban government officials as OD sites. OD sites are found in the open spaces between groups of slum dwellings, on the borders of railway lines or roads, down gullies or on rocky outcrops where construction is impossible, or on the edge of a settlement beyond the current edge of the slum. To allow any form of privacy they need by definition to be isolated, hidden, and unlit, making them unsafe for women and children.

Sanitation programming still tends to happen without full awareness of the role of gender and other aspects of identity in constraining people from accessing sanitation. The effects on women and girls of lack of sanitation are well known; these include health problems and psychosocial stress (Sahoo *et al.* 2015). Pregnancy, menstruation, and menopause and ageing create additional challenges during women's life cycles. Gender inequality creates additional issues. For women, and in particular women in overcrowded, impoverished urban areas, lack of sanitation facilities creates physical insecurity and vulnerability to VAW, including harassment, rape, and assault.

Recent scholarship has emphasised the cross-cutting nature of poverty, caste, religion, and other aspects of identity, which intersect with gender to shape women's experiences of inadequate sanitation (Carrard *et al.* 2013). Women and children face unavoidable risks when they relieve themselves, creating a range of problems and causing acute psychosocial stresses. Because of the state of many PTs in slums, women may see OD as a more appropriate choice. As Deepa Joshi *et al.* (2011, 102) write, 'What is experienced as lack of appropriate sanitation is defined significantly by where one lives'. Distant, open ground may seem more appropriate than spaces closer to home (Truelove 2011), but also a better option than a filthy, insecure PT.

In the next section, we give brief details of our research: locations, participants, and methods.

Our research

Mapping the research locations

An estimated 40 per cent of the population of Pune live in the city's vastis (Government of India 2011, 5), or slums, and in Jaipur, the figure is 16 per cent (PRIA 2014, 11). The study was done in three whole slums (Kathputli, Kalakar, and Lal Khan), and Swamion ki Basti (a slum pocket – that is, a small section of a big slum) in Jaipur, Rajasthan; and 11 slum pockets in Pune, Maharashtra (Ambedkar Nagar, Khadda Vasti, Birasdar Nagar, Gosavi Vasti, Laxmi Nagar, Lokamanya Nagar, Ganesh Nagar, Samartha Nagar, Rajiv Ghandi Nagar, Gulab Nagar, and Jaibhim Nagar). The locations for our research were selected with the help of NGOs working in the respective cities.

Due to lack of space we cannot describe the geography of each of these slums in full in this chapter, but we will focus briefly on a few examples, to enable readers to build up a picture of some of the key issues faced by partici-pants. Some slums are in the heart of the city. Others are far out, in peripheral locations. Slums can be 'declared' or 'undeclared'.[2] Many do not have roads, but stone and concrete slab walkways. Open drains are common. The housing pattern varies, with houses made of plastered or unplastered brick and con-crete floors and tin roofs, to rooms of tin covered with tarps or jute sacks. Some slums are electrified. Individual household latrines are almost unknown; some households built IHLs for women and girls, but these were rare.

Kathputli is the oldest slum in the city of Jaipur, at the city centre, with heavy traffic and a varied housing pattern from houses made of poorly mor-tared brick with tarpaulins or jute sacks instead of roofs to houses of plastered brick and concrete floors, with tin roofs. The land the slum occupies is pub-licly owned, although this is disputed. It is home to 5,000 people but has PTs in only one neighbourhood, with ten seats for men and ten for women. People here have household taps and public taps for water. Also in Jaipur, the slum of Kalakar is home to around 2,000 people. The area is north of the city centre and some houses have permanent construction, although many have dirt floors. The houses are very small and much activity goes on in the lanes between them. The sewerage system is a network of open drains. The PTs in the settlement are not in use because their construction was never completed.

In Pune, Ambedkar Nagar is a big city centre slum, home to around 10,217 people. It is a declared slum with private land ownership. Some people have private taps, and there are PTs with a caretaker, which the residents can use for a fee. There is an estimated one PT to every 500 people. In contrast, the small slum pocket of Khadda Vasti in Pune is home to 25 families – of around 111 people – who did not leave five years ago when the slum was evacu-ated. They now live in makeshift shelters on the footpath. There is no water or sanitation, and people practise OD in a space near the railway station. In another undeclared slum in Pune, Samartha, the land is privately owned and located on a hill. It is home to around 1,513 people. It has private drinking water connections, but only one PT located downhill, which is far away and in a filthy condition. There is an estimated one PT to every 1,000 people. Some families have constructed individual household toilets but others have to practise OD in a space on the hill. Finally, in the slum pocket of Ganesh Nagar, home to an estimated 427 people on another hillock in Pune, a tanker brings water every day for which women have to pay Rs 10–20 'incentive' to the tanker driver. There is no sanitation, and dwellers use an OD space located adjacent to the slum area.

In urban India, government provision of sanitation has taken various forms over the years. In some cases local governing bodies have given public land to NGOs for the building of pay-for-use facilities. In other cases, PTs have been built but they have far too few seats, no access to water, and their construction quickly crumbles. While some of these toilet blocks have caretakers, this was unusual in the slums we studied.

Research methods and participants

In our research, we used focus group discussions (FGDs) to give us basic familiarity with each settlement, its amenities, and women's experiences of sanitation-related violence. Women participants for FGDs were gathered by the NGOs working in those areas; some were engaged in NGO activities (like self-help groups) while others were not. They tended to be married women in their middle age, although newly married and elderly women also participated. These FGDs drew women from a variety of caste/ethnic/religious and socioeconomic groups. We also interviewed women selected from FGDs who were willing to talk in greater depth about their experiences and emotions.[3,4]

We aimed to interview across socioeconomic and geographic conditions in each study site.

All the locations we studied had a mixed caste and class composition. A total of 112 women participated in our research: 58 in Jaipur and 54 in Pune. Eighty-nine of the 112 (79 per cent) were aged between 18 and 45. Sixty-seven of the 112 women were totally uneducated. Women in Pune were roughly three times more likely to have had some formal education than women in Jaipur (12 compared to 34). The majority of women who had ever received education in Pune had been in school for between eight and ten years, while the picture was more varied over the whole spectrum in Jaipur.

Women were classified as either married (79 of 112), widowed (18), deserted (one) or unmarried (11). While all women do unpaid domestic work within the home, 39 of the 112 stated that this was their only work (expressed in our research as 'homemakers'). The rest worked outside their homes for money, providing informal urban labour. Twenty were domestic workers in the homes of better-off families, 16 did home-based work to produce small-scale goods or services, and 11 – all located in Pune – were wastepickers. Other occupations mentioned by relatively few women were construction work, working for an NGO, entrepreneur, dancer, government, *Anganwadi* worker (providing primary health care for pregnant women and young children), student, and beggar.

Caste/ethnic/religious identities are very important in these communities. As we will show, membership of different caste/ethnic/religious communities is a key factor in explaining women's experience – and perceptions of – sanitation-related VAW. The majority of women – 46 in Jaipur and 38 in Pune – were Scheduled Caste, a category including many communities identifying as Dalits, Chamars, Mahars, Nats, Rajnats, and others. Together they are a traditionally poor and stigmatised caste group. A small minority in both contexts were Muslim (seven women in Jaipur and three in Pune). The remaining participants (five in Jaipur and 13 in Pune) fell into the categories of Other Backward Caste, General, Scheduled Tribes, Denotified Tribes, and Nomadic Tribes.

Everyday violence and psychosocial stress: sharing our findings

Four significant themes regarding gendered violence and psychosocial stress emerged from our analysis: first, the theme of slum geographies and types of sanitation space, focusing on those who had no access to IHLs and had to use either PTs, or resort to OD; second, forms of harassment and assault and the experiences of women from different caste/ethnic/religious communities; third, mothers' fears for their daughters; and finally, coping mechanisms. In this section, we offer an analysis of our key findings according to these four themes. For each of these themes, we found that cross-cutting differences in identity – including gender, caste, religion, age, and others – affect women's experiences within the slum environment. The physical environment of the slum including its location, physical features including the natural environment, and infrastructure are all critical, as are social relationships.

Slum geographies and conditions of sanitation spaces

Availability of sanitation spaces was largely determined by the physical and social geography of the slums, and the investment in infrastructure that had been made by government, NGOs, and slum-dwellers themselves. Most of the slums on the outskirts had OD spaces, and those that were centrally located had PTs. Few households could afford IHLs. In some slums, defecation had to happen along the highway in full view of passersby, and/or on open ground without cover.

PTs

In Jaipur, all four slums had PTs, although only one – in Swamion ki Basti – was in useable condition. It had a caretaker, water, and was relatively clean. It cost INR 1 (US$0.02) to use. Another PT in Kathputli was built for the lowest caste group in the slum by a foreign donor, not far from a public tap. Women living nearby declared that the women's PTs were too filthy to be used:

> I had intended to use the PT, but two days after it is cleaned, it is too dirty to be used. (Interview, Jaipur, 3 January 2014)

In another location, Ambedkar Nagar, in Pune, there were five toilet blocks that were in poor condition. Only one of the five toilet blocks here was seen by participants in our research as in a useable condition, due to an on-site caretaker.

Wastepickers in Ambedkar Nagar had a better opinion of PTs over other users. Most said they were well-maintained, although not all thought positively about the facilities. Another woman, who is a domestic worker, from the same slum felt differently:

> The PTs are very dirty. Women eat tobacco and spit in the corners. They use the toilets to dump their sanitary napkins. Seeing all this, I once vomited when I used the toilet. Since then I prefer to avoid going in there if I can. I usually use the toilet in the houses that I work in as a domestic worker or a place of worship where such a facility exists. Otherwise, I prefer the open spaces near my *vasti*. (Interview, Pune, 18 November 2013)

The filth of the PTs in this slum was due to no running water for flushing, and no proper disposal for sanitary pads. Water had to be carried from home or obtained from a single outdoor tap near the toilet. The toilet use was timed, from 6 am in the morning until 11 am at night. Despite the poor state of the toilets, users were charged a fee of R1 per use. Affordability was a concern for women using PTs, and particularly so in situations like this one where payment was per use, rather than per month.

Many women in Pune slums chose to use OD sites because they judged the available PTs to be unsafe and filthy. Most were poorly lit, and the floors were wet and slippery, making them unsafe, especially for elderly, disabled, or pregnant women. The design of PTs, however well-intentioned, sometimes contributes to gender-related risks. For example, one PT had partial walls so daylight could enter and electricity be saved; however, women felt threatened by the possibility of men peeping over the walls and light at night was insufficient for women to feel safe.

Where PTs had women's toilets on the top floor (men's on the ground), women's vulnerability increased because of stairs and landings that were occupied by men drinking or playing cards. At least three slums had liquor stores situated near PTs that had broken, unlockable, or absent doors. One woman particularly mentioned the traumatic experience of looking at sexually graphic graffiti in the Pune slum of Laxmi Nagar, mentioned earlier. Because of the graffiti, she avoided defecating until absolutely necessary.

The opening times of PTs matters very much to women's safety, too. Even if women have access to a PT they feel they can use, they will have to go out in the open if they need to relieve themselves between 11 pm and 5 am. If a PT is only open during the day, the need to work will affect women's ability to use it. In Pune, working women left home by 8 am, and wastepickers even earlier. For these women, this means waiting to defecate later in the day, skipping morning household chores, or going for OD if they are too far from a PT.

OD sites

In Pune, OD sites contributed to creating risk and vulnerability for women because they were at a distant location from women's homes, and had characteristics contributing further to risk: located in scrubland and forests with undergrowth, at the side of railway lines and canals, and on hillsides and erosion gullies. OD sites were usually poorly lit or not at all. Several women narrated instances when steep, slippery sites led to broken legs, and railway tracks led to death. Lokmanya Nagar was located on one of the busiest roads in the city, had no PT, and hardly any open space for defecation.

OD sites often harbour snakes, pigs, insects, and other animals. A Scheduled Caste woman in Ganeshnagar-P narrated the menace of mosquitoes: 'They bite you all over' (interview, Pune, 15 October 2013). Another Scheduled Caste (Dalit) woman, who has now been able to afford an IPL, recalled:

> When I was a girl, my older sister and I went out for OD in the dark. I heard nothing until a dog bit me full in the face. I screamed and went into shock. My sister had to carry me home. For months I could not go out to the OD ground. (Interview, Jaipur, 9 January 2014)

Achieving privacy is impossible. In Kathputli, the OD place was across a dirt lane, busy with foot traffic that ran between the slum habitations and the OD ground. Avoiding anyone in order to get there was impossible at virtually any time of day. Being seen defecating was unavoidable as well – no plant growth existed to hide behind. Similarly, in the slum of Ganesh Nagar, OD simply had to be done along the highway in full view of passersby. Being watched or seen was a constant source of stress. A Scheduled Caste (Dalit) woman from Ganesh Nagar said:

> The defecation site is very close to the road, and therefore there is always a possibility that someone might be passing by. We have to keep looking in every direction for the passersby. Whenever we see someone approaching, we have to stand up, and then sit again when they are gone. (Interview, Pune, 10 October 2013)

When men came near the OD sites, women and girls said they either stood up, or tried to hide their faces, for example with scarves. Another Scheduled Caste (Dalit) woman said:

> We are always eagerly waiting for the evening ... If a male acquaintance sees you, it is so embarrassing when you meet him the next time. You can't keep your head down; you have to keep watch, so this is unavoidable. (Interview, Pune, 10 October 2013)

Yet the lack of privacy in OD also means that any attack is likely to be witnessed. One 40-year-old Muslim woman said, 'If I shout, someone will come running' (interview, Jaipur, 28 January 2014).

Violence, harassment, and caste dynamics

Sanitation-related VAW and sexual harassment was a constant threat to all women and girls, regardless of their caste/religion/ethnic identity, and regardless of whether they were using OD sites or PTs. This reality resulted in women consciously making decisions to minimise risk. However, for those who lack appropriate sanitation, what might be considered a 'normal' level of risk avoidance is simply not possible.

In our research, we heard of VAW and harassment that took both verbal and physical forms, and as one Jaipuri young woman told us, 'Looking is also harassment' (interview, Jaipur, 2 February 2014). In both Jaipur and Pune, women reported instances of harassment faced either by themselves or by other women known to them. Forms of harassment reported included men watching women during OD, perched in treetops, water tanks, and inside canals. They took pictures. A young Scheduled Caste (Nat) woman expressed her feelings this way,

> Teasing and watching are too normal to get worried about. It just happens. That's all. (Interview, Jaipur, 10 February 2014)

For her, harassment had become normal; since it was a usual occurrence, she had rationalised it by persuading herself that women should not fret over it.

Men do more than look; two women from Jaipur told us inappropriate comments were daily occurrences. In the Jaipur slum of Lal Khan, the OD main entrance was a hangout for young men. Young women and girls told us that they never answered back or noticed the loiterers in any way, but it was stressful just to pass by them. One young woman said that she used a short cut to the OD place in order to avoid them. Men also played cards along one perimeter of the OD place. A woman living on the periphery said that she kept an eye out for anything suspicious.

Women with children were also harassed. A wastepicker in Pune said,

> People who live on the footpath, don't like this [children defecating there], and they won't allow us to do it, if they see us. Also, people who clean the roads won't allow it. But there is no other place for children to defecate. (Interview, Pune, 19 February 2014)

Women reported that girl and boy children faced many of the same risks and harassment as adults.

While harassment was common, reports of sexual assault (including male masturbation) were few. In Ganesh Nagar, women specifically mentioned men staring and masturbating in front of them while they defecated. The worst incidents of VAW mentioned in our research were a rape in Jaipur, and an attempted rape in Pune. The woman who had undergone the attempted rape narrated the incident to us in detail. She observed:

> This place is very unsafe. It doesn't mean that nothing will happen in the future, just because it hasn't happened yet. Women always face a threat of being raped. (Interview, Pune, 10 October 2013)

We believe sexual assault was under-reported, due to the stigma attached to it. Sometimes we were being given accounts which indicated women were not willing to openly discuss instances of sexual assault. An example is that two women in Jaipur simply said a man 'stood' in front of them. The trauma of assault was compounded by community silence on the topic and women's lack of freedom to speak about it to each other, let alone to policymakers, planners, or researchers like us. For example, with bitterness, a 20-year-old Scheduled Caste woman related the story of how – when she was 15 and newly moved to the settlement as a bride – a man came and 'stood' in front of her. She shouted at him, and he ran. She continued, 'I did not tell my husband; I did not want to start a fight'. She concluded in anger:

> Even now, no one tells each other anything! How are we [women] to know what is going on [what to be afraid of]? (Interview, Jaipur, 5 February 2014)

Our interviews reflected this lack of information. We began asking women in Jaipur if they were certain of any sexual assaults occurring. Their response was to reply: 'No, but we know it happens in different places' (interview, Jaipur, 7 February 2014).

Intersectional perspectives: difference among women

A very important and striking finding of the research was the extent to which belonging to a majority community in the slum reduced women's risk of male harassment and violence.

In Jaipur's slums, women of dominant castes claimed that they felt no fear, faced no trouble, and had little experience with harassment. This enabled these women to put distance between themselves and other women's experiences and fears in the settlement.

An upper-caste woman, who was in a minority in the slums, told us how insecure she felt living among 'Dalits', and how she feared for her daughter's safety because of them. Women from that community presented the opposing perspective: they said they did not see a threat from 'other' men, since they saw 'their' men protecting them against sanitation-related violence. In Kalakar in Jaipur, women not belonging to the dominant Kalbelia[5] sub-caste were taunted by groups of Kalbelia boys, who played at the entrance of the OD place. However, Kalbelia women were apparently exempted from harassment: none of them reported experiencing it. In Ambedkar Nagar, in Pune, women said the local political representative had 'fixed' the 'outsiders', i.e. men not local to the area, thereby controlling VAW in the slum. 'Women' is a category that masks multiple differences, so we need not be surprised that caste and community relations presented a division.

Age and stage in the life cycle also created difference in gendered experiences of risk. Women reported that children of both sexes faced some of the same threats as adult women. Age and gender intersect to create particular risks for pre-pubescent and pubescent girls and whether they went for OD or used a PT, many women expressed particular fear for their daughters, rather than themselves. Women were especially concerned about their daughters' safety if they were physically or mentally challenged. Some women reported only letting daughters go for OD at night.

Women also expressed fear of their daughters having an illicit relationship when out visiting the OD site. In a traditional community where high value is placed on chastity before marriage, this is a very real fear. Women in all three Jaipur study sites mentioned that girls and boys met clandestinely at the OD place. A woman in Kathputli-J, who was one of the few upper-caste women we interviewed, told us,

> We had two young daughters, and I did not want them to go in the open any more. So I said to my husband that we will have to build our own toilet, even if we have to cut short on some other things. So when we built this house, we compromised on some other things. We did not build a kitchen counter immediately. But we built the toilet. (Interview, Jaipur, 29 January 2014)

For this woman, her family's minority, upper-caste position in the community made her daughter's safety her priority, and she accompanied her everywhere. She herself had not recovered from an incident when she was followed on her way to defecate.

Regardless of caste status, women said they did not allow their pre-teen and teenage daughters go for OD without them. As a mother lamented, 'once you lose your reputation, it is gone forever' (interview, Jaipur, 28 January 2014). A Scheduled Caste (Bhat) girl in Kalakar-J told us that if her mother cannot leave her current task then she has to wait before going out. A 20-year-old Scheduled Caste (Dalit) girl in Kathputli-J explained how different life was in the slums from life in the suburbs:

> When I am at my brother's house [in the suburbs], I am not afraid to walk on the street or go anywhere. (Interview, Jaipur, 9 February 2014)

In contrast, in the settlement, she was afraid of harassment, and never left the house except with her parents. Whether the fears were their own or their parents' projections, the result was a lack of freedom for teen girls in our study settlements.

The impact of unmet sanitation needs on physical, mental, and emotional health

The impact of having to restrain and control urges to defecate or urinate because of lack of safe, clean, and accessible sanitation facilities has a severe toll on health, in addition to numerous infections contracted from using filthy facilities.

A detailed inquiry into illness was not in the scope of our study, but women complained of skin infections, diarrhoea, urinary and reproductive tract infections, nausea, vomiting, and other illnesses. Mental and emotional health is affected as well as the more obvious and immediate threats to physical health. Sanitation affects all areas of women's and girls' lives, compromising their ability to work, but also their wider social well-being and relationships. For a woman in Pune, the stress of OD affected her sexual relationship with her husband as she was constipated most of the time. She reported that he suspected her of having an affair, due to her lack of interest in sex.

When we talked to women we tried to ensure we were discussing not only their current experience but also asking about their experiences over time. While the hazards associated with ODs and use of poor PTs were many, some were not constant, affecting some women due to health issues – for example, a need to rush out due to diarrhoea, or the urge to urinate more during pregnancy. Other hazards increased for all women and girls at particular times, for example during particular times of day when boys were gathered around OD sites, and taunting women who went there; or seasonal, as when monsoon rains made OD grounds so disgusting that women reported trying to defecate only every other day.

Our research brought out the multitude of psychosocial stresses that women face due to unsafe, inadequate, or absence of sanitation facilities. Women's stress and struggles around violence-free sanitation varied across a spectrum: from preoccupation with safety to the normalisation of harassment. Women mentioned feeling stress, trauma, shame, anxiety and guilt, embarrassment, and violation.

Experiences of psychosocial stress varied from woman to woman, depending on gender, caste, degree of poverty, age, and marital status. These aspects of personal identity shape women's experience but this is also shaped by the geography of the slums, with their specific characteristics of location, topography, and infrastructure, and the kinds of sanitation facility available to women. The issues also varied according to health and seasonality.

Women's coping mechanisms and strategies to effect change

Following Jo Rowlands (1997, 13), we wish to focus on the relational dimensions of women's power, as these hold the key to our original question: 'If gendered violence is symptomatic of power inequalities in society, then how do those inequalities manifest themselves in women's psychosocial stress and translate into women's decisions about where to relieve themselves?' Women are immersed in multiple relationships that determine the degree of harassment, fear of attack, and comfort when it comes to OD and PTs.

Our research showed the extent of stresses around sanitation but also highlighted women's resourcefulness and pragmatism, strategising to reduce their fear and discomfort. Coping with threats formed a part of women's everyday emotional lives. Remarks like 'What can we do?' and 'We have no choice' give insight into the degree of normalisation of women's fears surrounding OD and PTs. They also may be understood as women's feelings of helplessness around the issue of inadequate sanitation and its associated risks.

We found that women and girls feel they have to take responsibility for, or keep silent about, incidences of harassment. Social pressure means women and girls are under strain to preserve their reputations based on their behaviour outside their homes, and we found women blamed men from other communities for the risk, insecurity, violence, and harassment they feared and experienced.

A crucial point is that women themselves are more likely to analyse their experiences in terms of inter-communal harassment or violent acts committed by 'outsiders' than finding common ground with other women. We found women in our research showed little hesitation pointing out caste/sub-caste groups that engaged in harassment, but sexual assault was always attributed to an outsider. This may be because women were reluctant to name someone in their small communities; but it also suggests that men outside community sanctions seized opportunities to assault when they presented themselves. Notably, in both Pune and Jaipur, women's triumphant responses to attackers were against outsiders. Women related how their husbands discouraged their involvement in conflicts and women expressed suppressing an urge to confide in their husbands about experiences of violence.

Individual and household-level strategies

Women's greatest exercise of power lies at the most intimate scale: that of bodily control. In response to these issues, women and girls have developed strategies and coping mechanisms to deal with the challenges of sanitation in the slums. The most common way of coping is developing 'body discipline' (that is, trying to control bodily functions so that urination and defecation were as infrequent and safe as possible). Going out accompanied by other women, or husbands, also ensures women are safer than they are on their own by reducing vulnerability to accidental injury, and from violence and harassment. The ultimate goal women mentioned to solve the problem was being able to leave the group of people dependent on public sanitation or OD, by constructing and owning an individual toilet.

Women everywhere were knowledgeable about the safest times to go out for defecation. In order to avoid needing to go at other times, bodily discipline was much discussed. This was achieved by eating less at night, avoiding too much food and drink, avoiding spicy food, and using anti-diarrhoeal tablets to stop bowel function when necessary. Echoing the sentiments of others, a woman from Samarth Nagar in Pune told us:

> In case of upset stomach I either take a medicine, or eat something cold – like curd or ice-cream – to avoid going during the night. (Interview, Pune, 9 October 2013)

This woman said that she followed these preventive measures whenever there was no one to accompany her to the defecation site. A common individual coping mechanism reported was to go with a group of women either in the daytime or with husbands or other male household members at night. Some women wanted their husbands along; some husbands insisted on accompanying their wives. This reduced the risk of accidents. However, because it also reduced the risk of attack or harassment, this coping mechanism is simultaneously a strategy to challenge and reduce violence now and in the future. Yet as an action that takes place on the level of individuals and their households, it has limited scale and impact.

If we look at the struggle for sanitation as a struggle over sanitation 'resources' (that is, a safe, private, hygienic facility that is constantly available to those who need it), gendered negotiations around the safe use of OD and PT sites were to the disadvantage of women, while men were relatively privileged. Women's double burden of homemaker/caregiver and paid employee was illustrated in the lives of the women we spoke to. Many women faced greater or specific stress due to their specific needs to get out of the house for work, or took advantage of jobs with toilets even at reduced wages.

Without the protection of a husband, widows faced more physical insecurity, but married women recounted that their husbands set limits on their movement, time spent going for OD, and time of day of going out. Household gender relations were not necessarily antagonistic, however. Existing dangers meant a woman could successfully ask her husband to accompany her to the PT or OD ground.

Some husbands also responded to their wives' requests for IHLs for themselves or daughters.

Women's preferred solution to the stress of inadequate sanitation was to build IHLs. For most of the slum-dwellers in Pune and Jaipur, access to an IHL was financially out of reach. Existing IHLs were in either wealthy households or in the homes of those with disabilities or illness. In Jaipur, most often it centred on a pre-teen daughter and the need to build it before she got much older. Young women and girls were most at risk of VAW and harassment and the risk of attack created the need for women to accompany daughters to toilets or OD. This was a stressor not only because of their fear for their daughters, but also because of the time that it took from paid work and household chores.

Despite the risks faced by women and girls, male household members did not always immediately see the benefit of a household latrine. In Lal Khan, Jaipur, where women did piecework or worked outside their homes, two households reported building toilets, so that they could gain time for paid work. Two newly married young women who had grown up with IHLs fought with their husbands and in-laws to argue the need to build an IHL, and toilets were built in both cases.

Yet low rates of income, job insecurity, and land tenure insecurity played significant roles in decisions not to build. Women in Pune spoke frankly: 'We do feel like building our own toilets but the space too is not our own' and 'It's a vicious cycle since we don't have assured land titles, we cannot build toilets. Moreover constructing toilets is very expensive'.

Lack of space to build and the lack of drainage were other major hurdles reported.

Private or public building of IHLs across slums is not likely given financial and spatial constraints, unless city governments commit to investing in sewerage systems. That leaves PTs as the cost-effective option, but PTs are already 'magnets' for those who wish to harass or attack women and girls.

Individuals can fight for their own interests: 'I always fight back', said a Scheduled Caste (Rajnat) woman in Jaipur said (interview, 9 February 2014). Women may also intervene on behalf of each other, on an individual basis; another Scheduled Caste (Dalit) woman in Jaipur said she chased away a boy harassing a girl, but she did so without telling her husband who would have scolded her for interfering.

Finding solutions at scale in the slums: possibilities and constraints

Accounts of women's empowerment emphasise the role of collective action in increasing the 'power-to' of the individual so that it becomes part of the larger 'power-with' of the group (Rowlands 1997).

Where caste, sub-caste, or slum solidarity was strong, our research found that women did gather courage to counter harassment in a tough way: 'We are able to shout and beat men up if we are in bigger groups', said a woman from Ambedkar Nagar (interview, Pune, 29 November 2013). A group of women in Kathputli-J and wastepickers in Ambedkar Nagar did exactly that, and brought the man to the police station. Women also 'carry stones and masala [spice] along so that if some such incident were to take place we can take care of ourselves', said a woman from Ganesh Nagar (interview, Pune, 14 October 2013). This was echoed by other women from Birasdar and Ambedkar Nagar.

Inter-caste solidarity between women was also present. A story of inter-caste assistance came from an 18-year-old Scheduled Caste (Bhat) girl who told us boys from the Jogi community had helped her:

> My friend and I went for OD. As we were squatting there, some [Scheduled Caste] Jogi boys shouted to us that a man was watching us and we should run away. Then those Jogi boys beat the outsider up. I told my parents, and I told my sister about the nightmares I had afterwards. (Interview, Jaipur, 4 January 2014)

Most of the stories women told us were about the dangers of girls speaking to boys outside their sub-caste, but her story was of aid between sub-caste groups.

The idea of collective action to demand sanitation was mentioned in the research: wastepicking women demanded PTs in the 1990s after violence against women going for OD galvanised them. Yet PT technology on its own has not solved the issue of sanitation in the slums. PT sustainability is a key concern given the scale and levels of need, and the inequalities in social relationships that perpetuate risk and lack of access. Gendered sanitation-related violence is as much about inequalities as technical solutions. Some women will continue to use PTs regardless, but many others return to OD with all its associated fears and threats.

Collective action to advocate for more and improved PTs and to create communities which work together to maintain them is a challenge. Women in the slums differ not only in age from each other, but in caste, relative poverty, and other aspects, creating inequality between them. Tensions between groups play out in gendered ways, including – as we saw in our findings – VAW and harassment.

The possibilities for women joining forces across caste groups in Jaipur seemed to us to be small; communities in the city appeared to be viciously caste-divided, as evidenced by a riot in one of the slums during our interview period. Little community support in Jaipur was evident against sanitation-related violence or for the provision of sanitation, although occasionally women from multiple castes worked together in egregious cases of harassment.

In comparison, the situation in Pune was different: a mixed-caste group had demanded PTs from the city, and got them in 2000, although clearly this provision did not meet needs, as our research shows.[6] Wastepickers in Pune seemed to draw strength and motivation from being part of a union. The respondent who told us this said at the time the union was founded and collective action began, there were no toilets in the *vasti*, and women often faced violence. Men used to hide in the bushes and grab women when they went for defecation, so a group of women came together to demand a PT. As a result, a few PTs were constructed by the Municipal Corporation (interview, Ambedkar Nagar, 19 November 2013).

However, given the many ways that slum populations were distinct (that is, according to degrees of poverty) and chose to distinguish themselves (e.g. via notions of belonging and 'othering' playing out as caste pride/prejudice), solidarity over sanitation issues seems to us to – at least currently – be unlikely.

Conclusion

We believe that research like ours, that focuses on the common ground and differences in women's stories about sanitation add nuance to mainstream policy debates and can assist in the development of policies that will lead to sustainable sanitation. Women's own stories demonstrate how complex inequalities of gender, caste, and other aspects of difference create a need for appropriate sanitation that keeps children, adults, and households safe from sanitation-related ill health and stresses.

Notes

1. In Pune, NGOs involved were: SAMYAK, Kagad Kach Patra Kashtakari Panchayat, Khelghar, Bahujan Hitay, Pune Project – Jeevak; in Jaipur: Participatory Research in Asia (PRIA – Jaipur).

2. 'Declared slums' are those recognised by the government and therefore eligible for some basic services such as water and sanitation, as opposed to 'undeclared slums', which are considered to be illegal by the government and therefore not deserving of any basic services.
3. FGDs and interviews were not recorded; instead, notes were taken and then typed. Typed notes were coded by recurring themes and analysed by the authors. The research was approved by the Texas A&M Institutional Review Board and the Institutional Review Board of Chest Research Foundation, Pune.
4. The Swacch Bharat Abhyian – Urban (Clean India Mission – Urban) guidelines suggest that one seat in a PT is enough to serve the needs of 35 people. For women, the norm is 25 to a seat and for men it is 35 to a seat (Government of India, Swacch Bharat Mission – Urban Guidelines).
5. The Kalbelia caste traditionally earns its living through dancing, which is in particular demand for tourist performances in Jaipur.
6. For further information on the wastepickers union in Pune, see www.kkp-kp-pune.org/ and www.swachcoop.com/.

Notes on contributors

Seema Kulkarni is a senior team member with the Society for Promoting Participative Ecosystem Management (SOPPECOM) on issues of gender resources and livelihoods. Email: seemakulkarni2@gmail.com

Kathleen O'Reilly is Professor of Geography and Presidential Impact Fellow at Texas A&M University. She has studied water and sanitation in rural and urban India for 23 years, with a focus on the gendered impacts of inadequate sanitation and related psychosocial stress. Her work has been funded by the National Science Foundation and the Bill & Melinda Gates Foundation.

Sneha Bhat works with Society for Promoting Participative Ecosystem Management (SOPPECOM) as Research Associate, on the issues of gender, water, and livelihoods.

References

ActionAid (2013) *Women and the City II: Combating Violence Against Women and Girls in Urban Public Spaces – The Role of Public Services*, http://www.action-aidusa.org/sites/files/actionaid/women_and_the_city_ii_1.pdf (last checked 6 June 2017)

Bapat, Meera and Indu Agarwal (2003) 'Our needs, our priorities: women and men from the slums in Mumbai and Pune talk about their needs for water and sanitation', *Environment and Urbanization* 15(2): 71–86

Carrard, Naomi, Joanne Crawford, Gabrielle Halcrow, Claire Rowland and Juliet Willets (2013) 'A framework for exploring gender equality outcomes from WASH programmes', *Waterlines* 32(4): 315–33

Doron, Assa and Robin Jeffrey (2014) 'Open defecation in India', *Economic & Political Weekly* 49(49): 72–78

Government of India (2011) 'Census of India: Alphabetical List of Towns and Their Population Maharashtra', http://www.censusindia.gov.in/towns/mah_towns.pdf (last checked 6 June 2017)

Hirve, Siddhivinayak, Pallavi Lele, Neisha Sundaram, Uddhavi Chavan, Mitchell Weiss, Peter Steinmann and Sanjay Juvekar (2015) 'Psychosocial stress associated with sanitation practices: experiences of women in a rural community in India', *Journal of Water, Sanitation and Hygiene for Development* 5(1): 115–126

Joshi, Deepa, Ben Fawcett and Fouzia Mannan (2011) 'Health, hygiene and appropriate sanitation: experiences and perceptions of the urban poor', *Environment and Urbanization* 23(1): 91–111

Kwiringira, Japheth, Peter Atekyereza, Charles Niwagaba and Isabel Günther (2014) 'Gender variations in access, choice to use and cleaning of shared latrines; experiences from Kampala Slums, Uganda', *BMC Public Health* 14: 1180

McFarlane, Colin, Renu Desai and Steve Graham (2014) 'Informal urban sanitation: everyday life, poverty, and comparison', *Annals of the Association of American Geographers* 104(5): 989–1011, available at http://dro.dur.ac.uk/12431/1/12431.pdf?DDD14+dgg0cm1 (last checked 6 June 2017)

Osumanu, I.K. and E.A. Kosoe (2013) 'Where do I answer nature's call? An assessment of accessibility and utilisation of toilet facilities in Wa, Ghana', *Ghana Journal of Geography* 5: 17–31

PRIA (Society for Participatory Research in Asia) (2014) *Schemes for urban poor*, unpublished pamphlet

Rowlands, Jo (1997) *Questioning Empowerment: Working with Women in Honduras*, Oxford: Oxfam GB

Sahoo, Krushna C., Kristyna R.S. Hulland, Bethany A. Caruso, Rojalin Swain, Matthew C. Freeman, Pinaki Panigrahi and Robert Dreibelbis (2015) 'Sanitation-related psychosocial stress: a grounded theory study of women across the life-course in Odisha, India', *Social Science & Medicine* 139: 80–89

Scouten, M.A.C. and R.W. Mathenge (2010) 'Communal sanitation alternatives for slums: a case study of Kibera, Kenya', *Physics and Chemistry of the Earth*, Parts A/B/C 35(13-14): 815–22

Truelove, Yaffa (2011) '(Re-)Conceptualizing water inequality in Delhi, India through a feminist political ecology framework', *Geoforum* 42(2): 143–52

CHAPTER 3

Mainstreaming gender in the WASH sector: dilution or distillation?

Julie Fisher, Sue Cavill and Brian Reed

Abstract

The way women's issues have been conceptualised and acted on in the context of water, sanitation, and hygiene (WASH) has changed over the past four decades. The discourses and trends in development studies – from the Women in Development approach of the 1970s to Gender and Development in the 1980s – were mirrored in the WASH sector. The WASH sector has contributed to, and been shaped by, debates on women's needs and, latterly, on gender perspectives based on a combined argument for equity and efficiency. In addition, in the last decade, the WASH sector has developed its own distinctive initiatives, such as menstrual hygiene management and, recently, specific WASH considerations relating to gender-based violence. This paper assesses whether the result of this sector-specific response has been a dilution or distillation of gender issues. It concludes that the WASH sector has not disregarded the goals of women's empowerment and gender equality; rather, it has contributed to understandings of how resources – such as infrastructure and services – underpin that empowerment. This allows an important recognition of the value and impact of WASH-sector priorities and actions for the wider well-being of women.

Keywords: Women; gender; water; sanitation; equity

Introduction

The Sustainable Development Goals (SDGs) mark an increased level of commitment to water, sanitation, and hygiene (WASH). By 2030, Target 6.1 aims to 'achieve universal and equitable access to safe and affordable drinking water for all', whilst Target 6.2 aims to 'achieve access to adequate and equitable sanitation and hygiene for all, and end open defecation, *paying special attention to the needs of women and girls and those in vulnerable situations*' (United Nations 2016).

The wording of Target 6.2 draws attention to the needs of women and girls, rather than the generic need to consider gender or 'everybody', and is specific in relation to sanitation and hygiene, rather than water. This raises certain important issues. Does Target 6.2 echo development theories rooted in

http://dx.doi.org/10.3362/9781788530866.003

the 1970s, reflecting both a desire to assist people to meet their basic needs as well as to promote the potential of Women in Development (WID) perspectives current at that time (Moser 1993) And/or, is Target 6.2's wording based on the notion that the sanitation and hygiene needs of women and men differ (with attention to menstrual hygiene implicit), whereas the need for water does not? A third possibility is that this reflects greater awareness and recognition of the gendered differences in need for sanitation and hygiene – which also exist for water. Does this target on sanitation represent an important change in direction for the WASH sector, or have we been here before? Is the implication of this that a mainstreaming approach to gender[1] in the WASH sector has failed?

This chapter examines these issues through the lens of an historical review. It follows the intertwined threads of ideas about women, gender, and WASH, and the kinds of development and humanitarian programming that have resulted, relating these to key global events and core publications. The authors are an interdisciplinary group, and we will draw on our expertise in both social science and water and sanitation engineering to identify trends from the last four decades of theory and practice. This chapter reflects the language and priorities of both of these disciplines.

Women, gender, and WASH: what do we know?

WASH provision is widely accepted today to have important consequences for women and girls, impacting on their daily wellbeing and status in society, affecting their education, health, income, and safety (Fisher 2006a). Examples are:

- Responsibilities for household water collection and management are intrinsically linked to women and girls' domestic role in the household, e.g. cooking, cleaning, laundry, childcare, and care of the sick and elderly (Boserup 1970).
- The effects of collecting water on schooling do not impact uniformly on children's education (Doyle 1995). A one-hour reduction in the time spent walking to a water source increases girls' school enrolment by 18–19 per cent in Pakistan, and 8–9 per cent in Yemen (Koolwal and van de Walle 2010). Furthermore, the unavailability of effective latrines for girls in schools, with facilities for appropriate menstrual hygiene management, has been shown to impede girls' school educational achievement (Sommer *et al.* 2015).
- Carrying heavy water loads, on the head or back by women and girls, is associated with exhaustion, pain, discomfort, and musculo-skeletal damage (Hoy *et al.* 2003).
- Women report that water collection can be a significant source of chronic stress due to pressure to return home quickly, e.g. because of outstanding household tasks, anxiety about children left at home alone,

or husbands' suspicions of the time spent away from the home (Henley *et al.* 2014). More recently, attention to psychosocial stress and sanitation has been investigated in a number of settings (Hirve *et al.* 2015; Stevenson *et al.* 2012).

- Although access to WASH is not the root cause of gender-based violence, inadequate provision and location of facilities can make women and girls more vulnerable to harassment and assault (House *et al.* 2014).
- As WASH becomes more readily available, it is plausible that women will use the time freed up for income-generation or can create income dependent on water supply (Joshi and Fawcett 2001; Koppen 1997; Touré 1998).
- Alternatively, time saved by WASH can be used by women for their own development and empowerment, e.g. 'taking part in community activities or spending time with friends and family ... boosting personal growth and feelings of self-worth' (Oxfam internal document, April 2017). In Morocco, Florencia Devoto *et al.* (2012) found that people did not use the extra time generated by household water connections for productive activities; the extra time and the decrease in stress levels (and inter/intrahousehold water-related conflict) related to water collection increased households' self-reported happiness. The time saved did not increase the time family members spent generating income, through working or starting a business, or the time that children spent studying but households used the time for leisure and social activities (*ibid.*).
- WASH in health-care facilities is critical to maternal and neo-natal health (Velleman *et al.* 2014).
- Women with disabilities are made particularly vulnerable if they are unable to access WASH (Jones and Reed 2005) and lower-caste women may be excluded even if projects are meant to be gender sensitive (Joshi and Fawcett 2001).

It is clear from the examples that both human biology and gender roles and relations result in women engaging with both water and sanitation in ways that are different from men. This was formally recognised at a global level in the 1992 Dublin Principles (ICWE 1992),[2] with Principle 3 being 'Women play a central part in the provision, management and safeguarding of water'.[3]

Ideas about women and gender have been addressed in WASH narratives over time in different ways. The context for both the WASH sector-specific focus on women, and the evolution of the field of WID through to Gender and Development (GAD), has been a range of broader changes in development and humanitarian thinking and action, notably a focus on appropriate technologies in the 1980s, social development in the 1990s, 'gender mainstreaming' in the wake of the United Nations (UN) Fourth Women's Conference at Beijing in 1995 (UN 1996), and emphases on equity and inclusion from the 2000s. The sector has moved from seeing women as beneficiaries, to an instrumentalist focus on women's inclusion in WASH, with women taking an active part in the provision of water, as committee members or mechanics. Interest in women and gender issues in WASH was sparked by the experiences of the International Drinking Water Supply and Sanitation Decade (IDWSSD), which ran between 1981 and 1990 (Narayan 1995).

These ideas evolved into a gendered approach, which looks at gender roles and relations and from there typically focuses on women's role in the household and empowering women. However, latterly the WASH sector has moved back towards more women-centric and individualist approaches.

Analysing trends in papers at the WEDC Conference

To gain a sense of the changing priorities for WASH and women, we found it useful and interesting to analyse the proportion of papers presented at the annual International Conference of the Water, Engineering and Development Centre (WEDC)[4] relating to this topic (see Figure 1). We flag up many examples of these papers in our account here.

The WEDC Conference is a mixed academic and practitioner conference, covering technical and socioeconomic aspects, so reflects both thought and action in the WASH sector. Although the first conference was held in 1973, it was not until over a decade later that the first paper relating to women appeared, in 1984. By the end of the IDWSSD, the number of papers containing the word 'women' in the title peaked at 16 per cent (five out of 31).

Since then, the proportion of titles with 'women' in the title has fallen, but some of this can be explained in terms of shifts in thinking within the field, leading to changes in terminology. First, the drop in titles with 'women' were followed by an increase in use of the term 'gender', and more latterly, the terms 'equity' and/or 'inclusion', which could either be following general trends (from WID to GAD), moving away from a technical focus on women's

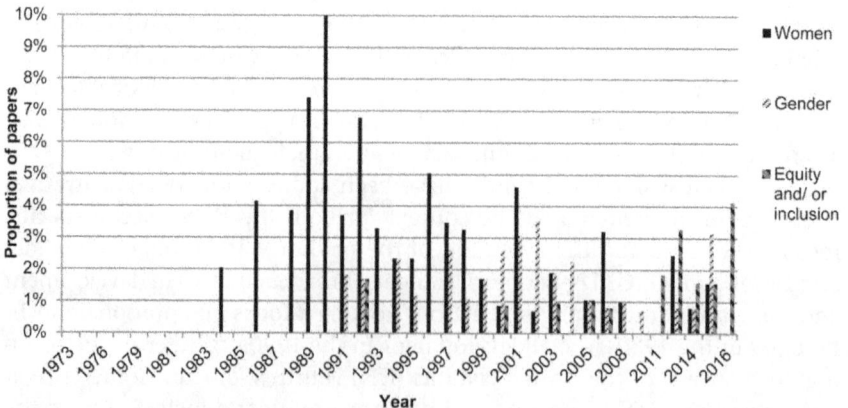

Figure 1. Proportion of WEDC conference paper titles containing relevant 'gender' keywords (the data for 1990 goes off the scale, to 16 per cent).

needs and roles to a greater appreciation of social aspects based on either wider development trends or the direct experience of WASH projects, or signal a move to focus on social identities including gender, ethnicity, or caste (focused on either separately or together as intersecting differences creating complex disadvantage).

The average proportion over the last ten WEDC conferences was 4 per cent (of about 120 papers presented annually) of these three categories ('women', 'gender', and 'equity/ inclusion'). This is an underestimate, however, as some authors do address gender issues or conduct gender analysis, but this is 'mainstreamed'– that is, integrated into their work and not flagged up explicitly in the title. Examples of words used to implicitly denote gender-disaggregated data or methods focusing on household and community dynamics are, for example, 'participation'/'participative' or 'community'. Papers using these two terms have held steady over the life of the conference, comprising about 8 per cent. However, the emphasis on gender issues has evolved in these papers over the years, reflecting increasingly sophisticated understandings of differences in community and the gendered dynamics of participation (Guijt and Shah 1998).

With these trends in mind, in the next sections we offer a chronological account of what lay behind them.

Evolving perspectives on women and gender issues over time

The 1970s: WID

Women's experiences, perceptions, and roles in WASH became an important area of focus from the early 1970s, in the lead-up to the First UN World Conference on Women in 1975. Debates in this period reflected the influence of second-wave feminism in international development and was based on proliferating studies of gender differences in roles and the connections between these roles and unequal power relations. In particular, the work of feminist anthropologists and feminist economists received increasing attention and led to increasing acceptance of the ideas that women were being either 'left behind' by development, and/or included on unequal terms and exploited by the prevailing Western development model. A growing body of research led to increasing pressure from feminists inside and outside international development organisations for governments and international institutions to respond.

From the 1970s, a range of WID policy approaches (Moser 1989) evolved from a common understanding that women's experience of development was different from men's (Rathgeber 1990). Parallel to the development of WID approaches, another very important policy approach of the era that is relevant to how women and gender are addressed in WASH was the Basic Needs Approach (International Labour Organization 1976), which sought to ensure that people had their basic needs met (including WASH). This approach, like the majority of WID approaches, focused on women's work, and justified a focus on women in WASH programming in two ways. First, these approaches emphasise the importance of the gender division of labour in shaping the particular roles of women and men in households and communities and recognise the need for a gender analysis in order to understand women's gendered WASH-related roles and responsibilities. Second, both WID and the Basic Needs Approach often portrayed women as more hardworking, caring, and responsible than men, and thus better able to meet their families' basic needs. Both these points led to the conclusion that focusing on women in WASH programmes could be expected to improve the effectiveness of projects, and providing water would specifically benefit women in their caring role.

WASH projects developed in the mid-1970s confirm the tendency to view the collection of water as intrinsically linked to women's role as household managers (Palmer 1977). This was a step forward from WASH programming in which services are typically directed at households, where it was assumed that resources and services are pooled equitably according to need. WASH interventions informed by WID perspectives went further, to focus on support to women in their reproductive role – now more often referred to as 'unpaid care work' (Esquivel 2014) – that is, domestic activities such as, water collection, cooking, cleaning, laundry, childcare, caring for the sick and elderly, and ensuring the family's health.

Using WID analyses of gender roles, improved WASH, specifically water, programmes were intended as a strategy to ease women's work burdens, enabling them to become more independent economically and participate more actively in community development activities (*ibid.*). Yet WID has been critiqued for seeing women as an untapped resource in WASH projects and programmes (Elmendorf and Isely 1981; van Wijk-Sijbesma 1985, 1987). Evidence offered at WEDC Conferences (including these early papers: Dotse *et al.* 1995; Libatique 1994; Shrivastava 1992) showed that participation of women could be used to provide skills, resources, labour, and cost-recovery in service delivery for improved projects.

Studies at this time often also focused on the potential of appropriate technology to reduce women's reproductive workload within the household (Elmendorf and Buckles 1980; Kalbermatten *et al.* 1980). Evidence suggested that the sustainability of water programming – always a challenge – is secured where communities have local ownership, and demand for services as well as the resources, information, and incentives to manage them (Roark 1980). Women featured in an instrumental capacity, as a cost-effective means to improve services, thereby contributing to the perpetuation of gender as a 'bolt on' to any agenda.

The 1980s to 1990s: a focus on inequalities

A critique of WID grew out of a concern with the impact of class, gender, and social relations for development processes. This criticised both the Basic Needs Approach and WID for their non-confrontational approach (Rathgeber 1990).

They were seen as failing to challenge existing patterns of inequality or question the division of labour within households, instead focusing on how women could better be integrated into development initiatives. Both approaches were critiqued for their focus on the transfer of appropriate technologies as a sole solution to complex issues which required addressing more holistically. Appropriate technologies were presented as the solution to women's domestic workloads, and the time saved was depicted as time to be spent specifically on income generation. This critique called for a different approach that focused on the politics of inequality. Both a Women and Development (WAD) approach and a GAD approach were mooted as successors to WID (*ibid.*). It was GAD which gained currency and signalled a shift from including women in existing unequal models of global development to a focus on gender, race, and class-based inequalities and an emphasis on women's right to set the development agenda (Moser 1989).

GAD was acknowledged to be an essentially political approach which was particularly concerned with issues of equity and social justice. GAD proponents argued that the household was a site of struggle, with competing rights and conflicting interests between male and female household members (Sen 1990). A GAD perspective, therefore, would aim not only to change the design of WASH interventions, but to re-examine the gendered power relations, social structures, and institutions that determine women's position in society relative to men. Projects informed by this aim focused on the need to ask women themselves for their own definitions of empowerment, to support women to organise themselves for collective decision-making, and to gain more economic resources, but also to provide space for movement building and to ensure women in the global South became a powerful and effective political voice. This approach aimed to move the outputs of development programmes and projects away from women as beneficiaries or women as actors, to a broader agenda for social change. Water projects could be seen by some as an entry point for this social engagement.

In 1995, the UN Fourth World Conference on Women was held in Beijing, entitled 'Action for Equality, Development and Peace'. This conference produced the Beijing Declaration and Platform for Action (UN 1995), which talked about the right of women to equality with men throughout the whole life cycle. However, infrastructure and basic services, including water and sanitation, were not a major focus for Beijing.[5] The global publicity given to women and gender issues in 1995 was reflected in that the choice of theme of World Water Day that year, designated by the UN General Assembly, was Women and Water.

Throughout the 1990s, and beyond into the 2000s, the WASH literature focused on women's empowerment in programming (Ivens 2008). However, the WASH rendition of empowerment was narrower than the GAD understandings, tending to focus on the levels of individual, household, and collective empowerment that are necessary to ensure sustainable WASH programming (El Katsha and Watts 1993). The shift to the language of empowerment helped to focus programming on the opportunities that participation offers to women's empowerment processes, and this potentially offers scope to build a sense of individual self-confidence and attain the skills and resources necessary for self-reliance. In addition, programmes promoting women's participation and leadership challenged traditional perceptions of women's status, skills, and capabilities. In the WASH research of the time, there were many examples where women were trained as handpump caretakers, even if on a voluntary basis (Baden 1993; Regmi *et al.* 1999; Wakeman 1995), and other examples of potentially empowering programme choices which may have had a primary aim of sustainability but could also result in other positive effects for women, as individuals and as a collective marginalised group.

The influence of evolving understandings of development and global movements for gender equality is reflected in WASH-sector research and programming priorities of the time. One year after Beijing, in 1996, the WELL Resource Centre for Water, Sanitation and Environmental Health (known as WELL) was established. The WELL Guiding Principles (WELL 1998, 2) state that 'People matter more than science', and that 'all too often the perspectives and roles of women are ignored or undervalued. We need to understand demand for services from women, men, and children across all social groups before selecting suitable approaches and technologies'. WELL was at the forefront of a number of equity and inclusion issues in WASH, through its research, teaching, collaborations, and evaluations.

At the end of the IDWSSD in 1990, the Joint Monitoring Programme for Water Supply and Sanitation (JMP) was launched by the World Health Organization and UNICEF, to monitor WASH progress at the country level. By presenting disaggregated statistical evidence each year, the JMP demonstrates that the poorest and most disadvantaged people continue to be left behind with regard to access to improved WASH. Findings focusing attention on inequalities based on wealth and geography have latterly been complemented by attention to specific identity groups, such as people with disabilities, and analysis of age groups (e.g. WASH in Schools) have been augmented by greater understanding of the fact that individuals experience different inequitable outcomes that change over the life course.[6] In the same year, the Water Supply and Sanitation Collaborative Council (WSSCC) was established, advocating for improved sanitation and hygiene for everyone, and facilitating local technical solutions for effective sanitation and hygiene provision (Wakeman 1995).

The 2000s: gender mainstreaming in WASH

The focus on gender mainstreaming that emerged from the 1995 Beijing Conference continued in the new millennium, slowly influencing WASH institutions and organisations. The need to ensure development and humanitarian organisations can deliver women's empowerment requires a focus on the culture and ways of working of the organisations themselves. In WASH, strategies included recruiting gender advisers to work with WASH specialist staff in a range of different ways, appointing 'gender champions' to raise the profile of gender issues among staff, and developing conceptual analytical frameworks, strategies, indicators, and other technical guidance to help staff incorporate gender equity issues into their work. WASH programming was adopting additional goals concerned with women and gender issues alongside the core aim of improving or enabling the provision of WASH infrastructure.

Attempts were made to mainstream gender in the Millennium Development Goals (MDGs) that framed global development from 2000 to 2015. At the start of the new century, the UN Millennium Declaration committed to reduce extreme poverty in its many dimensions. In relation to WASH, MDG 7, focusing on environmental sustainability, included a target to halve, by 2015, the total proportion of those without sustainable access to safe drinking water, with a target on access to basic sanitation added in 2002. Other targets focused on slums: Target 7.D was to achieve, by 2020, a significant improvement in the lives of at least 100 million slum dwellers. MDG 3, the Gender Goal, aimed to: 'Promote gender equality and empower women', but had only one target, to 'Eliminate gender disparity in primary and secondary education, preferably by 2005, and in all levels of education no later than 2015'.

Whilst the MDG target on water and sanitation [Target 7.C to halve, by 2015, the proportion of the population without sustainable access to safe drinking water and basic sanitation] did not explicitly focus on gender, action to integrate women's rights and gender equality into WASH continued, and in the year 2000 the Gender Water Alliance was established to promote equitable access to – and management of – safe and adequate water as a basic right for all, recognising this as a critical factor in promoting poverty eradication and sustainability. Also by the early 2000s, equity issues were becoming more routinely included in regional sanitation conferences including AfricaSan (in 2002)[7] and SACOSAN (in 2003),[8] addressing regionally specific challenges to the achievement of universal access.

In 2004, the Women for Water Partnership, involving 100 countries, was established to raise the profile of women in the sector. Partnerships of women's organisations and networks proved an effective way to promote voice and accountability for gender equality and women's empowerment at country, regional, and international levels. An example of a national analysis dating from the same period which informed bilateral aid decisions' action was the UK Government's Department for International Development's (DFID) Target Strategy Paper published in 2000. It recognised that:

> Women are highly dependent on basic transport, energy, secure shelter, and water and sanitation services to enable them to carry out their economic and social roles. Many of these are often poorly related to women's needs, significantly adding to the costs for women of carrying out their responsibilities and reducing the effectiveness and efficiency of public investment in these areas. Failure in design work to address

cultural considerations may severely constrain women's use of sanitation and other facilities. More gender-aware approaches will enable planners, engineers, and managers to bring important gains to economic and social development, as well as making an important contribution to reducing the burden on women. (DFID 2000, 18)

Started in the 1980s, DFID's Knowledge and Research (EngKaR) programme funded several research projects on gender issues in the management of water projects in the 2000s as well as a subsequent piece of DFID-funded research, entitled 'Gender Issues in the Promotion of Hygiene and Sanitation Amongst the Urban Poor' (2001–2004). This research resulted in a number of outputs intended to help water engineers understand gender issues, and how to apply this understanding to their work (Reed and Smout 2005).

In the 2000s, mainstreaming gender issues within WASH programming became an accepted norm, and conceptual tools and frameworks were developed to help with this. Brian Reed *et al.* (2007) offered an initial technical response to a social need through practical guidance for engineers, technicians, and project managers on how infrastructure can meet the needs of men and women.

At a global level, in 2004, the UN established an Advisory Board on Water and Sanitation, to galvanise global action on WASH issues. In 2005, as part of the Global WASH Campaign, the WSSCC established the Women Leaders in WASH programme to support women leaders in Africa to advocate for better services, with material such as 'For Her It's the Big Issue' (Fisher 2006). This highlighted the issues and problems women face, and the need to have women at the centre of decision-making and management of WASH services.

For water, the International Decade for Action 'Water for Life' (2005–2015) launched the UN Human Development Report (2006) of the same theme, arguing that poverty, power, and inequality – not water scarcity – are at the heart of the problem of supply. In November 2006, DFID recognised that safe and affordable water is a right for all. For sanitation, the International Year of Sanitation (2008) aimed to increase attention given to sanitation. The fact that inadequate sanitation affects women in very distinct ways, threatening their safety, privacy, and status, for example, in ways that do not affect men, was recognised more widely at this point (Brocklehurst and Bartram 2010; O'Reilly 2010). The eThekwine Declaration on Sanitation was made at AfricaSan 2008, recognising gender and youth and the importance of involving women at all levels of decision-making.

However, whilst the global agenda on gender was promoting empowerment and decision-making, a new strand appeared in the WASH sector: in 2002, the ground-breaking work of Hazel Jones and Bob Reed on 'water and sanitation for disabled people and other vulnerable groups'. Although its focus was quite specific, it demonstrated that a move to ensure WASH programmes resulted in accessible and inclusive services for all not just women (Jones and Reed 2005). This had a strong practical element, with clear design guidance as well as programming advice.

In the same vein, in the early 2000s, WELL produced a series of Briefing Notes and 40 fact sheets on a range of equity and inclusion issues including: school sanitation (Mooijman *et al.* 2004), disabled people's needs (Jones and Fisher 2005), putting women at the centre of WASH (Fisher 2004), gender (Fisher 2004), and HIV/AIDS (van Wijk 2003). Attention on sanitation broadened beyond women, with organisations such as IRC and UNICEF addressing issues relevant to children in schools (Reed and Shaw 2008). This development was mirrored with the topics being presented at the WEDC International Conference, with papers specifically on the needs of schoolchildren, menstrual hygiene management, and the needs of people with disabilities. These resonate with WID approaches that the physical provision of basic services is still required if socially excluded people are to benefit. Whilst the vision of women's empowerment is founded on women controlling sufficient resources to enable them to take decisions and actions in their lives (Kabeer 1995) through appropriate participation and engagement, the primary, core outputs of these WASH projects are physical infrastructure, not wider social change.

The 2010s: equity and inclusion

This decade has been characterised so far by the WASH sector 'pulling the scales from our eyes' with respect to the issues of equity and inclusion (Chambers 2012, 14) – that is, addressing issues of marginalisation and exclusion in order to ensure access to safe water and sanitation for all. This has played out in various ways, demonstrating the formal recognition and acceptance by the international WASH community of the importance of a rightsrather than a needs-based approach, and its varied impacts. In 2010, WaterAid produced its Equity and Inclusion framework (WaterAid 2010), and since then other agencies have followed suit. Notably, Juliet Willetts *et al.* (2010) reviewed the synergies between the MDG targets on gender and WASH, even though gender was – as discussed earlier – not a specific aspect of MDG 7.

In 2012, the first Special Rapporteur on the human rights to safe drinking water and sanitation linked the notion of stigma to WASH and brought issues of discrimination, degrading treatment, and privacy to the forefront (De Albuquerque and Roaf 2012). Furthermore, WASH for women and girls was a theme for a number of UN reports, including both the 2012 and 2013 World Development Reports (World Bank 2012, 2013) and, in 2015, the UN Water Report was entitled, 'Eliminating Discrimination and Inequalities in Access to Water and Sanitation' (UN Water 2015). In the same year, the UN General Assembly adopted a resolution on the human rights to water and sanitation. The Global Analysis and Assessment of Sanitation and Drinking-Water (GLAAS)   (see   http://www.who.int/water_sanitation_health/monitoring/investments/glaas/en/, last checked 6 June 2017) monitors whether countries recognise drinking water and sanitation as a human right in national legislation and reports on a country's commitment to reducing disparity, for instance the extent to which equity and inclusion considerations (e.g. population groups that are poor, live in slums or remote areas, or live with disabilities) are integrated into policies, plans, and budgets.

Significant recent publications by WSSCC are promoting attention to equity and inclusion across the life course, such as 'We Can't Wait' (WaterAid, Unilever, and WSSCC 2013) and 'Leave No One Behind' (WSSCC and FANSA 2016) – reflecting the focus of the SDGs on complex inequalities (de Roure and Capraro 2016). At the end of the MDG period, with the SDGs in sight, Working Groups were established (including one on Equity and Non-Discrimination) to propose WASH targets and indicators for global monitoring after 2015 (Satterthwaite 2012). In 2015, the SDGs were enacted, bringing this account full-circle to the point at which we started.

In addition, during this decade, the WASH sector developed work around women's gender-specific interests and needs. In particular, the concept of menstrual hygiene management became visible; menstruation and the particular needs of women that arise from it has until recently been absent from WASH debates – effectively, a taboo subject. The work of Sowmyaa Bharadwaj and Archana Patkar (2004) has acted as a catalyst for a very productive stream of work on this theme. Since then, menstrual hygiene management has been acknowledged as a vital concern, demonstrated by guidance manuals (e.g. House *et al.* 2012), and a plethora of research papers (as can be seen in Figure 2). Consideration to women's gender-specific concerns arising from female biology has now extended to WASH and the peri-menopause (Bhakta *et al.* 2014).

In different development and humanitarian sectors, the 2010s has so far been a decade in which the existence of gender-based violence, in particular sexual violence and violence against women and girls, has been much more widely recognised than before. In the WASH sector, 'Violence, Gender & WASH. A Practitioner's Toolkit', from Sarah House *et al.* (2014), takes a sector-specific perspective on a wider gender issue, looking at practical steps that WASH practitioners can take to reduce risks to vulnerable people.

Also over this decade, a life-course approach to programme design has become evident, and this enables specific attention to be given to groups of people made vulnerable by a range of factors. Examples are female heads of households, and their household members (Carolini 2012), people with disabilities, children, elderly people, or pregnant women. The specific interests and needs of women and girls require particular attention in the context of WASH in institutions such as schools and health facilities (Velleman *et al.* 2014).

New areas of study and action into the factors underpinning vulnerability of different groups are still emerging. For example, the WASH sector is slowly developing a better understanding of how gender identity, as well as sexual orientation, affect the use of facilities, including use of sex-segregated toilets by transgender people, as well as harassment of LGBTI children in school facilities (Coyle and Boyce 2015).

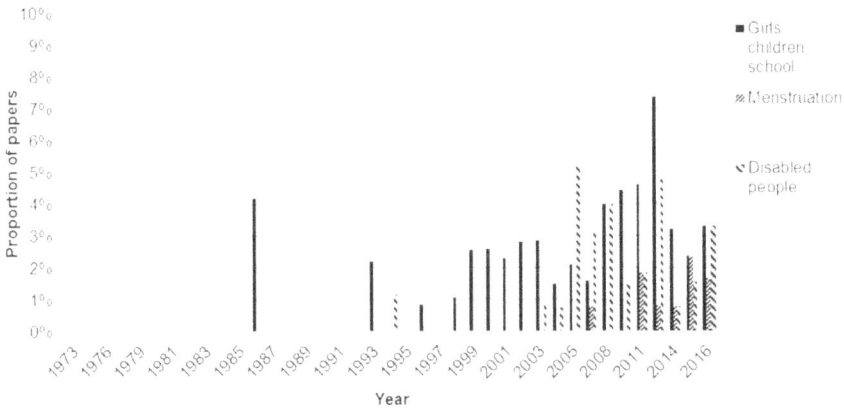

Figure 2. Proportion of WEDC conference paper titles containing relevant 'inclusion' keywords.

Looking back: dilution or distillation?

Tracing the parallel evolution of women and gender issues and WASH practice over the last four decades reveals a complex picture. Has the process of integrating women and gender into WASH resulted in a dilution of these issues, or a distillation of them? In this section and the following one, we examine what has happened, and look forward to what lies ahead.

It is clear that increased recognition has been given in WASH programming to the importance of gender identity, roles, and relations in achieving universal access to WASH. Beyond the focus on gender identity, progress is being made to understand the importance of multiple and overlapping identities of excluded people; some WASH services (such as water) are easier to provide equitably than others (such as sanitation). In line with the SDG commitment to 'Leave no one behind', WASH programmes are more alert to a variety of markers of difference: socioeconomic class, ethnicity, language, disability, income, and stage in the life cycle. People and issues that were once invisible (such as slum dwellers, disabled people, adolescent girls, and menstrual hygiene) are now incorporated into WASH programmes, as a result of the current focus in the sector on equity and inclusion.

These developments suggest a growing divergence between WASH-sector priorities and global approaches to gender equality and women's rights, as WASH has adapted approaches to meet its own identified sub-groups and sub-issues. The broad focus on WASH and women is being sub-divided into more nuanced themes, recognising that women are not a single homogenous group and that needs change over the life course. This does not indicate a neglect of women and WASH, but a more finessed understanding of individuals by the sector and their specific needs related to water and sanitation. The recognition that women have interests arising from multiple identities – that women's interests is a broader category than 'women's gender interests' – is not new in

GAD – it was recognised by Maxine Molyneux as early as 1985 – but the WID and GAD approaches to gender and women in development programming have focused on the gender aspects of their experience, focusing on advancing women's rights as a single category. By practically working with women on the ground means WASH professionals see complex inequalities playing out and excluding particular individuals. 'Gender' has been disaggregated into increasingly specific categories of social exclusion by the WASH sector for pragmatic reasons related to the delivery of water and sanitation services.

The actual work undertaken by the WASH sector in communities is more nuanced. Instrumentalist arguments were typically used in relation to women and gender. Examples discussed earlier included targeting women in their existing gender roles as carers, or ensuring efficient maintenance of WASH facilities. This instrumentalisation of gender issues does appear to have reduced at a policy level and been replaced by arguments focusing on women's empowerment. However, the mainstreaming of gender into WASH programmes may have resulted in socioeconomic issues such as empowerment and representation being diluted by the need to physically deliver water and sanitation services. Complex, contextual social analysis is difficult to carry out and respond to in a meaningful way within the framework of delivering public infrastructure. However, this has been balanced by the distillation of the underlying gender and social inequalities into practical steps that the WASH sector can deliver successfully to the benefit of specific, recognisable groups. At a project level, indicators of WASH progress do not normally include issues of empowerment, but these issues are not diluted, just concentrated into practical steps that can be delivered successfully.

Looking forward

We know the importance of good goals, targets, and indicators in development, and in the SDGs, the indicators and their ability to deliver progress are all-important. WASH indicators of progress on the provision of WASH need to be chosen that do not just reflect delivery of infrastructure but make a real difference in enabling women's control of WASH resources – understanding this as an essential aspect of women's current and future empowerment. Empowerment indicators focusing on including women in water governance and maintenance were common in development work in the past – such as ensuring that a proportion of women were appointed to a WASH management committee (Dotse et al. 1995). The current trend towards indicators that make a real difference to women in their current gender role as household carers is important and starts the empowerment process from where women currently are. It is as least as valid from a gender equality and women's empowerment perspective as focusing on women's participation and leadership in infrastructure provision and maintenance, and is more valid from a WASH perspective as it works at the same time and spatial scale as infrastructure provision.

The indicators that are being developed for the SDGs align closely to women's needs as carers for households. Under SDG Target 6.1, indicator 45 is the 'percentage of population using safely managed water services … ', where 'households are considered to have access to safely managed drinking water service when they use water from a basic source *on premises*' (Sustainable Development Solutions Network no date). By setting the standard for water to be *an on-plot level of service*, the target is inherently and effectively addressing all the issues of the burden of water collection that disproportionally impact on women and girls, but without specifically mentioning this. Target 6.2 will be measured by 'percentage of population using safely managed sanitation services' (*ibid.*), with the type of *household* latrine being assessed. Both these WASH targets will be disaggregated by urban or rural location, but not by gender as the basic unit of assessment is the household. This potentially creates problems for monitoring from an equity perspective. Whilst female-headed households will be included in the target, intra-household inequalities could lead to problems accessing sanitation services at the household level.

Conclusion

This chapter started with an assessment of the WASH SDGs; it is worth comparing these with the gender Goal 5: to 'Achieve gender equality and empower all women and girls'. Whilst the targets for Goal 5 do cover empowerment, decision-making, and education, Target 5.4: states: 'Recognize and value unpaid care and *domestic work* through the *provision of public services*, *infrastructure* and social protection policies and the promotion of shared responsibility within the household and the family as nationally appropriate' (emphasis added). This is a recognition that basic infrastructure provision continues to have a role in gender issues, although no infrastructure-related indicator has been proposed under Goal 5 (http://indicators.report/goals/goal-5/). The provision of WASH – and other basic resources needed for life – are fundamental elements in the empowerment of women and gender equality. The role of basic resources including WASH infrastructure should not be underestimated or forgotten by the women's movements in their activism and struggles to achieve empowerment of women and gender equality. All development sectors need to work together to empower women and attain gender equality, but they also need to work together to deliver basic services for all, developing sector-specific responses to global challenges. Women's movements need to call for empowerment *and* better sanitation.

Integrating gender perspectives by the WASH sector has been critical in their effort to 'leave no one behind'. The WASH sector has not disregarded empowerment; rather, it has recognised the vital importance of the role of infrastructure in that empowerment. The WASH sector does not have the tools to change society, but it can ensure that the provision of good basic infrastructure services is equitable. Gender issues are being distilled, not diluted.

Notes

1. Gender mainstreaming refers to the integration of gender analysis into all areas of planning and policy for development, as a strategy to bring about gender equality and support women's equal rights. It was taken up widely as a strategy in the wake of the UN Fourth Conference on Women in 1995.

2. Dublin Principles: part of the preparation for the UN Conference on Environment and Development in Rio de Janeiro in June 1992. *Principle 1: Fresh water is a finite and vulnerable resource, essential to sustain life, development and the environment.* Since water sustains life, effective management of water resources demands a holistic approach, linking social and economic development with protection of natural ecosystems. Effective management links land and water uses across the whole of a catchment area or groundwater aquifer. *Principle 2: Water development and management should be based on a participatory approach, involving users, planners and policy-makers at all levels.* The participatory approach involves raising awareness of the importance of water among policymakers and the general public. It means that decisions are taken at the lowest appropriate level, with full public consultation and involvement of users in the planning and implementation of water projects. *Principle 3: Women play a central part in the provision, management and safeguarding of water.* This pivotal role of women as providers and users of water and guardians of the living environment has seldom been reflected in institutional arrangements for the development and management of water resources. Acceptance and implementation of this principle requires positive policies to address women's specific needs and to equip and empower women to participate at all levels in water resources programmes, including decision-making and implementation, in ways defined by them. *Principle 4: Water has an economic value in all its competing uses and should be recognised as an economic good.* Within this principle, it is vital to recognise first the basic right of all human beings to have access to clean water and sanitation at an affordable price. Past failure to recognise the economic value of water has led to wasteful and environmentally damaging uses of the resource. Managing water as an economic good is an important way of achieving efficient and equitable use, and of encouraging conservation and protection of water resources.

3. The focus on women in the Dublin Principles, mentioned in the last section, is welcome; while the focus changed around the start of the 1990s from 'women' to 'gender'– at least at the level of the language used to describe policy approaches and programming – and a gender analysis needs to be the starting point of work in any community since gender relations vary according to context. However, critics have suggested that the shift from 'women' to 'gender' risks underestimating the importance of addressing specific issues that women experience in contexts of gender inequality, and that need to be prioritised. The term 'gender' also masks issues that relate mainly to women in a physical way, such as menstruation and child birth.

4. WEDC is one of the world's leading education and research institutes for developing knowledge and capacity in water and sanitation for lowand middle-income countries. WEDC is based in the School of Civil and Building Engineering at Loughborough University: http://wedc.lboro.ac.uk/ (last checked 3 April 2017).

5. The Beijing Declaration and Platform for Action Turns 20 notes low levels of resources allocated to sectors such as water and sanitation as a major challenge to the full implementation of the Platform for Action: https://sustainabledevelopment.un.org/content/documents/1776The%20Beijing%20Declaration%20and%20Platform%20for%20Action%20turns%2020.pdf (p. 53) (last checked 3 April 2017).

6. For further information, see www.wssinfo.org/ (last checked 3 April 2017).

7. AfricaSan, organised by the African Ministers' Council on Water is a pan-African political initiative intended to promote political prioritisation of sanitation and hygiene and attended by Ministers responsible for sanitation and the key agencies working in sanitation and water in Africa: www.africasan.com/ (last checked 3 April 2017).

8. The South Asian Conference on Sanitation (SACOSAN) is a government-led biennial convention held on a rotational basis in each SAARC (South Asian Association for Regional Cooperation) country, which provides a platform for interaction on sanitation. SACOSANs are intended to develop a regional agenda on sanitation, enabling learning from the past experiences and setting actions for the future: www.sacosanv.gov.np/sacosan (last checked 3 April 2017).

Acknowledgement

The authors thank the editor for her contributions, especially highlighting WASH issues and concepts that may not be familiar to the readership of the journal.

Notes on contributors

Julie Fisher Lecturer at the Water, Engineering and Development Centre (WEDC), Loughborough University, UK. Email: J.Fisher1@lboro.ac.uk

Sue Cavill is a WASH consultant.

Brian Reed is Lecturer in Water, Engineering and Development at Loughborough University, UK.

References

Baden, Sally (1993) *Practical Strategies for Involving Women as Well as Men in Water and Sanitation Activities*, BRIDGE Report No. 11, Brighton: Institute of Development Studies

Bhakta, Amita, Julie Fisher and Brian Reed (2014) *WASH for the perimenopause in low-income countries: changing women, concealed knowledge?* Briefing Paper 1909 at the 37th WEDC International Conference, Hanoi, Vietnam

Bharadwaj, Sowmyaa and Archana Patkar (2004) *Menstrual Hygiene and Management in Developing Countries: Taking Stock*, Mumbai: Junction Social, Social Development Consultants

Boserup, Ester (1970) *Woman's Role in Economic Development*, London: George Allen & Unwin. (Reprinted in 2007)

Brocklehurst, Clarissa and Jamie Bartram (2010) 'Swimming upstream: why sanitation, hygiene and water are so important to mothers and their daughters', *Bulletin of the World Health Organization* 88(7): 482–482

Carolini, Gabriella Y. (2012) 'Framing water, sanitation, and hygiene needs among female-headed households in periurban Maputo, Mozambique', *American Journal of Public Health* 102(2): 256–261

Chambers, Robert (2012) 'Equity and Inclusion: Pulling the scales from our eyes', in WSSCC (ed.), *Global Forum on Sanitation and Hygiene. Insights on Leadership, Action and Change*, Geneva: Water Supply and Sanitation Collaborative Council, 14–15

Coyle, Daniel and Paul Boyce (2015) *Same-sex sexualities, gender variance, economy and livelihood in Nepal: Exclusions, subjectivity and development*, Evidence Report No 109, Sexuality, Poverty and Law, Brighton: Institute of Development Studies

De Albuquerque, Caterina and Virginia Roaf (2012) *On the Right Track: Good Practices in Realising the Rights to Water and Sanitation*, Lisbon: Human Rights to Water and Sanitation, UN Special Rapporteur and ERSAR

de Roure, Sarah and Chiara Capraro (2016) 'Faith paths to overcome violence against women and girls in Brazil', *Gender & Development* 24(2): 205–218

Devoto, Florencia, Esther Duflo, Pascaline Dupas, William Parienté and Vincent Pons (2012) 'Happiness on Tap: Piped Water Adoption in Urban Morocco', *American Economic Journal: Economic Policy* 4(4): 68–99

DFID (2000) *Target Strategy Paper – Poverty Elimination and the Empowerment of Women*, London: DFID

Dotse, F., Mawuena, Nii Odai Laryea and Betty Yankson (1995) *Can rural women manage water?* 21ˢᵗ WEDC Conference, Kampala, Uganda, 1995: http://wedc.lboro.ac.uk/resources/conference/21/Dotse2.pdf (last checked 6 June 2017)

Doyle, Brendan A. (1995) 'Increasing education and other opportunities for girls and women with water, sanitation and hygiene', *Waterfront* UNICEF-Special Issue, August

El Katsha, Samiha, and Susan Watts (1993) *The Empowerment of Women: Water and Sanitation Initiatives in Rural Egypt*, Cairo: American University in Cairo Press

Elmendorf, Mary, and Patricia Buckles (1980) 'Appropriate technology for water supply and sanitation', *Appropriate Technology* 3: 1

Elmendorf, Mary L., and Raymond B. Isely (1981) 'Role of women as participants and beneficiaries in water supply and sanitation programs,' WASH Technical Report No. 11, December, Washington, DC: US Agency for International Development

Esquivel, Valeria (2014) 'What is a transformative approach to care and why do we need it?', *Gender & Development* 22(3): 423–439

Fisher, Julie (2004) *The Gender Millennium Development Goal. What water, sanitation and hygiene can do.* WELL Briefing Note 4, Loughborough: WEDC, Loughborough University

Fisher, Julie (2006) *For Her It's the Big Issue: Putting women at the centre of water supply, sanitation and hygiene*. Evidence Report, Geneva: Water Supply and Sanitation Collaborative Council (WSSCC)

Henley, Phaedra, Megan Lowthers, Gideon Koren, Pamela Tsimbiri Fedha, Evan Russell, Stan VanUum, Sumedha Arya, Regna Darnell, Irena F. Creed, Charles G. Trick and John R. Bend (2014) 'Cultural and socio-economic conditions as factors contributing to chronic stress in subSaharan African communities', *Canadian Journal of Physiology and Pharmacology* 92(9):725–32, doi:10.1139/cjpp-2014-0035. Epub 2014 Jul 7

Hirve, Siddhivinayak, Pallavi Lele, Neisha Sundaram and Sanjay Kamlakar Juvekar (2015) 'Psychosocial stress associated with sanitation practices: experiences of women in a rural community in India', *Journal of Water, Sanitation and Hygiene for Development* 5(1): 115–126

House, Sarah, Suzanne Ferron, Marni Sommer and Sue Cavill (2014) *Violence, Gender & WASH: A practitioner's toolkit. Making water, sanitation and hygiene safer through improved programming and services*, SHARE Consortium, http://violence-wash.lboro.ac.uk/ (last checked 6 June 2017)

House, Sarah, Therese Mahon and Sue Cavill (2012) *Menstrual hygiene matters. A resource for improving menstrual hygiene around the world*, London: WaterAid

Hoy, Damian *et al.* (2003) Low back pain in rural Tibet, The Lancet, 361(9353): 225–226, cited in Hazel Jones and Bob Reed (2005) *Water and sanitation for disabled people and other vulnerable groups: Designing services to improve accessibility*, Loughborough: WEDC, Loughborough University

Human Development Report (2006) *Beyond scarcity: Power, poverty and the global water crisis*, New York: UNDP, http://hdr.undp.org/en/content/human-development-report-2006 (last checked 6 June 2017)

ICWE (International Conference on Water and the Environment) (1992) *The Dublin Statement on Water and Sustainable Development* Dublin, Ireland, http://www.wmo.int/pages/prog/hwrp/documents/english/icwedece.html (last checked 6 June 2017)

International Labour Organization (1976) *Employment, Growth and Basic Needs: A One-World Problem*, Geneva: ILO

Ivens, Saskia (2008) 'Does Increased Water Access Empower Women?' *Development* 51(1): 63–67, doi:10.1057/palgrave.development.1100458

Jones, Hazel and Bob Reed (2005) *Water and Sanitation for Disabled People and Other Vulnerable Groups: Designing Services to Improve Accessibility*, Loughborough: WEDC, Loughborough University

Joshi, Deepa and Ben Fawcett (2001) *Water projects and women's empowerment*. 27th WEDC Conference, Zambia, http://wedc.lboro.ac.uk/resources/conference/27/Joshi.pdf (last checked 6 June 2017)

Kabeer, Naila (1995) *Reversed Realities: Gender Hierarchies in Development Thought*, London: Verso

Kalbermatten, John M., DeAnne S. Julius and Charles G. Gunnerson (1980) *Appropriate Technology for Water Supply and Sanitation*, Washington, DC: World Bank

Koolwal, Gayatri and Dominique van de Walle (2010) *Access to Water, Women's Work and Child Outcomes*, The World Bank Poverty Reduction and Economic Management Network, Gender and Development Unit Policy Research Working Paper 5302, Washington, DC: The World Bank

Koppen, Barbara van (1997) *Gender and water rights, Burkina Faso and Bangladesh*, quoted in Julie Fisher (2008) Women in water supply, sanitation and hygiene programmes', *Proceedings of the ICE: Municipal Engineer* 161(4): 223–229, https://dspace.lboro.ac.uk/dspace-jspui/bitstream/2134/9920/13/muen161-223.pdf (last checked 6 June 2017)

Libatique, Ruthy C.D. (1994) *Empowering women to manage watsan technologies*. 20th WEDC Conference Colombo, Sri Lanka, http://wedc.lboro.ac.uk/resources/conference/20/Libatiqu.pdf (last checked 6 June 2017)

Molyneux, Maxine (1985) 'Mobilization without Emancipation? Women's Interests, the State and Revolution in Nicaragua', *Feminist Studies* 11(2): 227–254

Mooijman, Annemarieke, Marielle Snel and Julie Fisher (2004) *The EDUCATION Millennium Development Goal: What water, sanitation and hygiene can do*. WELL Briefing Note 2, http://www. lboro.ac.uk/well/resources/Publications/Briefing%20Notes/BN%20Education.htm (last checked 6 June 2017)

Moser, Caroline (1993) *Gender Planning and Development: Theory, Practice and Training*, London: Routledge

Narayan, Deepa (1995) *The Contribution of People's Participation : Evidence from 121 Rural Water Supply Projects*. Environmentally Sustainable Development Occasional Paper Series; No. 1, Washington, DC: The World Bank, http://documents.worldbank.org/curated/en/750421468762366856/Thecontribution-of-peoples-participation-evidence-from-121-rural-water-supply-projects (last checked 6 June 2017)

O'Reilly, Kathleen (2010) 'Combining sanitation and women's participation in water supply: an example from Rajasthan', *Development in Practice* 20(1): 45–56

Palmer, Ingrid (1977) 'Rural women and the basic-needs approach to development', *International Labour Review* 115(1): 97–107

Rathgeber, Eva M. (1990) 'WID, WAD, GAD: Trends in Research and Practice', *The Journal of Developing Areas* 24(4): 489–502

Reed, Brian and Ian Smout (2005) *Building with the Community: Engineering Projects to Meet the Needs of Both Men and Women*, Loughborough: WEDC, Loughborough University

Reed, Brian, Sue Coates, Marie Fry, Sarah Parry-Jones and Ian Smout (2007) *Infrastructure for All: Meeting the needs of both men and women in development projects. A practical guide for engineers, technicians and project managers*, Loughborough: WEDC, Loughborough University

Reed, Bob and Rod Shaw (2008) *Sanitation for Primary Schools in Africa*, Loughborough: WEDC, Loughborough University

Regmi, Shibesh Chandra and Ben Fawcett (1999) 'Integrating gender needs into drinking-water projects in Nepal', *Gender & Development* 7(3): 62–72

Roark, Paula (1980) *Successful Rural Water Supply Projects and the Concerns of Women*, Washington, DC: Office for Women in Development, US Agency for International Development

Satterthwaite, Meg (2012) JMP Working Group on Equity and Non-discrimination Final Report, New York, Geneva: WHO/UNICEF Joint Monitoring Programme for Water Supply and Sanitation

Sen, Amartya (1990) 'Gender and Cooperative Conflicts', in Irene Tinker (ed.) *Persistent Inequalities: Women and World Development*, New York: Oxford University Press, 123–129

Shrivastava, Satya Sagar (1992) *Community, women and domestic water.* 18th WEDC Conference Kathmandu, Nepal, http://wedc.lboro.ac.uk/resources/conference/18/shrivastava.pdf (last checked 6 June 2017)

Sommer, Marni, Nana Ackatia-Armah, Susan Connolly and Dana Smiles (2015) 'A comparison of the menstruation and education experiences of girls in Tanzania, Ghana, Cambodia and Ethiopia', *Compare: A Journal of Comparative and International Education* 45(4): 589–609

Stevenson, Edward, Leslie Greene, Kenneth Maes, Argaw Ambelu, Yhenew Tesfaye, Richard Rheingans and Craig Hadley (2012) 'Water insecurity in 3 dimensions: An anthropological perspective on water and women's psychosocial distress in Ethiopia', *Social Science & Medicine* 75(2): 392–400

Sustainable Development Solutions Network (no date) 'Indicators and a Monitoring Framework: launching a data revolution for the SDGs,' http://indicators.report/indicators/i-45/ (last checked 6 June 2017)

Touré, Yanflé (1998) 'Boreholes mean business', *Waterlines* 17(8): 26–7, available at http://www.ircwash.org/sites/default/files/Toure-1998-Boreholes.pdf (last checked 6 June 2017)

United Nations (1996) *Report of the Fourth World Conference on Women, Beijing 4-15 September 1995*, New York: UN, http://www.un.org/womenwatch/daw/beijing/pdf/Beijing%20full%20report%20E.pdf (last checked 6 June 2017)

UN Water (2015) *Eliminating discrimination and inequalities in access to water and sanitation,* Geneva: UN-Water, http://hrbaportal.org/wp-content/files/UN-Water_Policy_Brief_Anti-Discrimination.pdf (last checked 6 June 2017)

United Nations (2016) 'The Sustainable Development Goals', https://sustainabledevelopment.un.org/sdgs (last checked 6 June 2017)

van Wijk, Christine (2003) *HIV/AIDS and Water Supply, Sanitation and Hygiene.* WELL Factsheet, http://www.lboro.ac.uk/well/resources/fact-sheets/fact-sheets-htm/hiv-aids.htm (last checked 6 June 2017)

Van Wijk-Sijbesma, Christine (1985) *Participation of women in water supply and sanitation: roles and realities*. Technical Paper No. 22, The Hague: IRC

van Wijk-Sijbesma, Christine (1987) 'Drinking-water and sanitation: Women can do much', *World health forum* 8(1): 28–33

Velleman, Yael, Elizabeth Mason, Wendy Graham, Lenka Benova, Mickey Chopra, Oona Campbell, Bruce Gorden, Sanjay Wijesekera, Sennen Hounton, Joanne Esteves Mills, Val Curtis, Kaosar Afsana, Sophie Boisson, Moke Magoma, Sandy Cairncross and Oliver Cumming (2014) 'From joint thinking to joint action: a call to action on improving water, sanitation, and hygiene for maternal and newborn health', *PLoS Medicine* 11(12): e1001771

Wakeman, Wendy (1995) *Gender issues sourcebook for water and sanitation projects*, Washington, DC: The World Bank and Water Supply and Sanitation Collaborative Council

WaterAid (2010) 'Equity and inclusion: A rights based approach', http://www.wateraid.org/what-wedo/our-approach/research-and-publications/view-publication?id=d98d98ad-b605-4894-97cf-0c7682e62b04 (last checked 6 June 2017)

WaterAid, Unilever and WSSCC (2013) *We Can't Wait: A Report on Sanitation and Hygiene for Women and Girls*, London / Geneva: WaterAid, Unilever Domestos, WSSCC

WELL (1998) 'The WELL Principles', http://www.lboro.ac.uk/well/about-well/well-principles.htm (last checked 6 June 2017)

Willetts, Juliet, Gabrielle Halcrow, Naomi Carrard, Claire Rowland and Jo Crawford (2010) 'Addressing two critical MDGs together: gender in water, sanitation and hygiene initiatives', *Pacific Economic Bulletin* 25(1): 162–176

World Bank (2012) *World Development Report: Gender Equality and Development*, Washington, DC: The World Bank, https://siteresources.worldbank.org/INTWDR2012/Resources/7778105-1299699968583/7786210-1315936222006/Complete-Report.pdf (last checked 6 June 2017)

World Bank (2013) *World Development Report: Jobs,* Washington, DC: The World Bank, https://siteresources.worldbank.org/EXTNWDR2013/Resources/8258024-1320950747192/8260293-1322665883147/WDR_2013_Report.pdf (last checked 6 June 2017)

WSSCC (Water Supply and Sanitation Collaborative Council) and FANSA (Freshwater Action Network South Asia) (2016) *Leave No One Behind: Voices of Women, Adolescent Girls, Elderly and Disabled People, and Sanitation Workers*, http://wsscc.org/resources-feed/leave-no-one-behindvoices-of-women-adolescent-girls-elderly-persons-with-disabilities-and-sanitation-workforce/ (last checked 6 June 2017)

CHAPTER 4

Mainstreaming gender in WASH: lessons learned from Oxfam's experience of Ebola

Simone E. Carter, Luisa Maria Dietrich and Olive Melissa Minor

Abstract

Within Oxfam, we continue to question how we could have better integrated gender equality in the Ebola response, and how to improve our gender mainstreaming in future emergencies. Why did gender mainstreaming in the Ebola response prove particularly challenging? How did the Ebola response differ from previous emergencies? What did we need to know to improve our response to the outbreak? Are there new ways in which we should approach gender mainstreaming? What lessons have we learned that we can carry forward in our work? Most importantly, what recommendations can we offer beyond those already provided in existing guidelines? In this chapter, we reflect on our experience as non-medical specialist practitioners involved in the response, to help us answer these questions.

Keywords: Gender; Ebola; WASH; gender mainstreaming; lessons learned; humanitarian

Introduction

This chapter draws on the experience of Oxfam and represents one of many efforts within Oxfam to capture the lessons from its Ebola WASH (water, sanitation, and hygiene) response. Despite the existence of comprehensive gender equality standards and a robust body of gender mainstreaming guidelines, enhancing women's participation in WASH emergency programming requires better, faster, and comprehensive community engagement and context analysis. The 2014–15 outbreak of Ebola Virus Disease in West Africa was an unprecedented global public health emergency; reaching capital cities, and infecting nearly 30,000 people (CDC 2014).

This chapter was written as a part of Oxfam's learning on its Ebola response. It focuses on the challenges our WASH teams faced in integrating gender in the Ebola response. Staff and community feedback reveals some interesting and important lessons from the experience. We share and reflect on these, and provide recommendations for improving gender mainstreaming in WASH in the event of future epidemics. In particular, we find that the use of generic

http://dx.doi.org/10.3362/9781788530866.004

gender mainstreaming approaches overlooked the differential ways in which Ebola affected women and men. While both women and men were equally likely to become infected revealed that there was gender parity in numbers of infections, male and female gender roles created particular chains of transmission. Women's role as caregivers was important, but so too were other gendered dynamics leading to infections. A more nuanced approach to gender may have allowed for more appropriate and meaningful opportunities to engage with women and address barriers to women's full participation in the Ebola response.

As authors of this chapter, we are drawing on a range of sources, from a review of literature to our own first-hand experiences as Oxfam staff at the time of the Ebola response. All authors were, at the time of the Ebola response, part of Oxfam's Humanitarian Support Team (HSP), each providing different support to Oxfam's Ebola programme. Simone Carter is an Epidemiologist and specialist in Public Health Promotion and Community Engagement, Luisa Maria Dietrich is a Gender Advisor; and Olive Minor is an Anthropologist and Public Health Promotion Team Leader. In addition, we draw on various sources of information from other staff, and from community members. Simone Carter (Carter *et al.* 2017a; Carter *et al.* 2017b) and Olive Minor (2014) held qualitative interviews and focus group discussions within communities affected by the Ebola outbreak, and Luisa Maria Dietrich (2015) carried out participant observation and semi-structured interviews with female community members, as well as leader and key informant interviews with Oxfam staff (Dietrich 2015).

An online survey conducted in December 2016 provided another major source of information for this chapter. Twenty national and international Oxfam WASH team members who had worked in the 2014–15 WASH-Ebola response offered their views on the biggest challenges for gender mainstreaming in WASH, and their recommendations for improvement. The survey asked WASH teams what gender mainstreaming goals they had or had not reached, and why. We asked about the types of support they needed, and whether they felt they had that support, and elicited suggestions on how we could better achieve gender mainstreaming goals within Oxfam and within future epidemic responses.

Oxfam WASH programmes and Ebola

Prior to the Ebola outbreak, Oxfam had over a decade of experience in WASH programmes in each of the Ebola-affected countries: Sierra Leone, Liberia, Mali, Senegal, and Guinea Bissau. In each country, WASH programmes had previously transitioned from humanitarian, post-conflict interventions, to long-term WASH programming. Interventions included innovative sanitation in Senegal and Liberia, Urban WaSH in Sierra Leone, and long-term WASH in IDP (internally displaced people) camps in Mali.

In the first months of the Ebola outbreak in Sierra Leone and Liberia, Oxfam country teams halted all existing programmes due to staff safety concerns.

Despite increasingly desperate alarms from Médecins Sans Frontières (MSF), the World Health Organization (WHO) did not officially recognise the Ebola outbreak as a public health emergency until 8 August 2014, when the disease reached the USA (MSF 2015). This delay in decisionmaking by the WHO contributed to uncertainty within Oxfam and other organisations regarding our potential role in containing the outbreak, as well as our ability to protect our staff. Despite previous experience with cholera, hepatitis E, and smaller Ebola outbreaks, Oxfam (along with many other organisations) struggled to define how to use our WASH expertise to address the growing epidemic. In October 2014, Oxfam's leadership made a decision to intervene, dedicating all available resources to address an epidemic that MSF had already declared out of control on 23 June 2014 (MSF 2014).

With our previous experience of cholera and Ebola in Africa, Oxfam had developed templates for typical WASH outbreak responses. Yet the scale of the 2014 Ebola epidemic required us to confront challenges and refine the critical role of Community Engagement and Public Health Promotion (CE-PHP) and WASH in health crises.

Oxfam rapidly developed a WASH-Ebola programme to respond to the outbreak, using a three-tiered approach focusing on Treatment, Containment, and Prevention.

1. Treatment focused on working in partnership with medical actors to provide WASH services and materials for Ebola Treatment Units/Centres,[1] Community Care Centres, and health posts.
2. Oxfam WASH teams supported Containment efforts through aiding country-specific surveillance programmes. In Sierra Leone, this included training and deploying Community Health Volunteers (CHVs) to conduct house-to-house messaging and surveillance; in Liberia, Oxfam supported contact tracing teams in addition to CHVs' houseto-house work.
3. Prevention involved CE-PHP teams to increase vulnerable communities' access to Ebola prevention information, services, and materials (including water and soap), while actively engaging community participation in improving prevention and treatment-seeking behaviour.

Oxfam's approach to CE-PHP uses a community-driven model, in which we create two-way dialogue with existing community and governmental bodies, and adapt our programming based on their feedback. This community-centred approach was the context in which WASH teams implemented gender mainstreaming. Here, we use Oxfam's definition of gender mainstreaming:

> a strategy which aims to bring about gender equality and advance women's rights. It aims to do so by taking account of concerns about gender equality and building gender capacity and accountability into all aspects of an organization's policy and activities, in order to contribute to a profound organizational transformation. Such activities may include policy

and programme development and implementation, advocacy, organizational culture and resource allocation. (Oxfam 2017, 40)

The following section gives a brief account of Oxfam's progress on gender mainstreaming in WASH programming, followed by a section offering key information about gender mainstreaming within Oxfam's Ebola response. We then outline some key challenges articulated by Oxfam staff regarding gender in our Ebola response; discuss how Oxfam could have addressed those challenges; and offer recommendations for the rapid implementation of gender mainstreaming in the event of future disease outbreaks. Lastly, we consider the implications of this approach for broader WASH interventions.

Gender mainstreaming in Oxfam's WASH programming

Throughout Oxfam's years of experience working in WASH, we have strengthened our commitment to mainstreaming gender equality and women's rights in our programmes, particularly though the creation of the first gender unit in 1984. Since, Oxfam has also developed a number of gender assessment tools to aid in programme design and implementation. In emergency settings, the latter has been particularly important in contexts with very little time to assess the social relationships and power dynamics that affect people's access to resources, including resources offered as part of emergency responses.

Over the years, Oxfam has developed a series of these strategic guidance and practical tools on Gender in Emergencies. These share the common aim of promoting gender equality in preparedness and response programming for all humanitarian interventions. Strategic guidance includes Oxfam's 'Minimum Standards on Gender in Emergencies' (Oxfam 2013) and '2016–20 Gender in Emergencies Strategy' (Oxfam internal document, 2016). This focused on five areas of work: delivering effective quality response through upholding gender equality and women's rights; campaigning for gender justice and women's rights; strengthening partnerships for women's rights; enhancing staff capacity and commitment on gender equality and women's leadership; and strengthening women's agency, voice, participation, and leadership.

The need to ensure all staff involved in Oxfam's humanitarian programming received essential information and support on gender issues led to the writing of a brief, commonsense guide, *A Little Gender Handbook for Emergencies* (Clifton 1999). The guide maps out concrete activities along the project management cycle as these relate to the different kinds of humanitarian response Oxfam undertakes, including WASH. In addition, Oxfam has also published theme-specific guidance that is relevant to WASH, such as 'Transformative Leadership for Women's Rights' (Kloosterman 2014) and 'Ending Violence Against Women' (Oxfam 2012).

At a minimum, typical gender-responsive WASH practice within Oxfam now includes using gender analysis tools and frameworks to gather and analyse sex and age disaggregated data, and identify vulnerabilities based on gender, age, and (dis)ability. Some programmes may include workshops to build shared understanding of gender-specific needs in water, sanitation, hygiene, and public health. Both capacity-building and programming aim to address structural inequalities and support gender justice, mostly at household and community level. In all programming, Oxfam seeks to ensure that equal numbers of women and men receive training, that women receive equal pay for equal work, and that women have opportunities for meaningful participation in community spaces.

Yet gender mainstreaming continues to be a challenge in large-scale first-phase emergency responses. The Ebola crisis posed particular challenges that led Oxfam staff to doubt the success of gender mainstreaming in the response. Despite our efforts, a narrow view of gender mainstreaming meant that men's and women's roles in disease prevention remained poorly understood, and women's participation in response activities remained limited.

What did we do? Oxfam's Ebola response through a gender lens

The authors of this chapter provided specialist advice from our particular disciplines, to strengthen context analysis and resultant programming. This work included helping WASH teams to better understand the social barriers to compliance with Ebola prevention and treatment messages in Liberia (Minor 2014); understanding the barriers and enablers to treatment-seeking and causes of high-risk practices in Sierra Leone (Carter *et al.* 2017a); specific gender roles within the context of the outbreak (Minor and Kanneh 2015); and the impact of Ebola on women and girls in Sierra Leone (Dietrich 2015).

Gender mainstreaming activities included supporting Ebola-related rapid gender assessments (UN Women *et al.* 2014; Taqi 2015), training and advising technical staff, and contributing to project proposals. In addition, staff were able to draw on our backgrounds in anthropology, gender equality, and epidemiology, to provide daily fieldbased support to international and national WASH teams in Liberia and Sierra Leone.

In the online survey of December 2016, Oxfam's WASH teams said that they felt able to meet the minimum requirements for gender mainstreaming in the first phase of the interventions. They highlighted how having nearly equal numbers of women and men on Oxfam's WASH teams in turn contributed to greater gender parity among the CHVs. Because families often prioritise boys' education over girls', WASH teams struggled to find equal numbers of literate male and female CHVs, but did eventually recruit mostly gender-balanced teams. From the outset, this was critical in creating gender-segregated settings in which women and men could speak openly with CHVs of the same gender.

Secondly, staff highlighted the importance of adapting hygiene kits to include menstrual hygiene products, to allow women and girls under quarantine to go through menstruation with dignity. WASH programmes distributed menstrual hygiene kits with small amounts of soap and sanitary napkins to women and girls. However, kit replenishment in areas that underwent repeated quarantines became difficult.

Staff also discussed the importance of outreach and engagement with female leaders. Several of the questionnaire respondents referred to working with female chiefs, Mami Queens (female community leaders), and women's groups. Activities often drew upon pre-existing groups like farming co-operatives, youth groups, and women's empowerment groups. However, this was mostly done later in the response, once women's participation had been identified as a major challenge in our programmes.

The online survey also asked about the primary source of gender-related information among WASH staff. All survey respondents cited the work done by the authors as gender specialist, anthropologist, and epidemiologist, as key sources for their context analysis. This additional support was cited by all respondents as improving understanding of gender and overall context and being able to influence the quality of Oxfam's WASH intervention. Other non-government organisations (NGOs) engaged similar in-house expertise during the response, highlighting the important role of internal cross-cutting and overarching advisors who can support teams in critical thinking, reframing questions, and using this information to develop more appropriate interventions.

Bearing in mind the attention given to resourcing on gender and social aspects of the crisis, it was striking that both staff and community members consulted for this chapter felt that women's meaningful participation in the crisis response was still lacking, and genderrelated challenges had not been effectively overcome to ensure programming reached its goals. Staff online feedback focused on the challenges discussed later.

Challenges in our Ebola response from a gender perspective

Challenges identified by staff focused on three main concerns. These were the militarised nature of this large-scale response to Ebola, in countries where health and other systems were struggling; the limited participation of women and other traditionally marginalised groups in the planning and implementation of the response; and the impact of a narrow gender mainstreaming lens on programme effectiveness, leading to a focus on women and unpaid care work at the expense of a wider approach incorporating the roles of men and boys. Below, we look at each of these challenges in turn.

Militarised responses in fragile contexts: the impact on women's participation

Ebola's context created particular challenges around governance and capacity to respond to a large-scale crisis involving a highly infectious disease. The scale and severity of the 2014 Ebola outbreak strained international and national capacities to deploy an effective response. While Oxfam is no stranger to providing WASH in militarised, fragile, and conflict-affected settings, the mobilisation of the military in response to Ebola in West Africa occurred on a new and different scale. This had serious implications for the treatment of traditionally marginalised groups, including women. As Oxfam's Gender Brief for Ebola (Dietrich 2015) pointed out, crises that involve the military are more likely to constrict women's participation.

In Sierra Leone, the Ministry of Defence organised a National Ebola Response Centre (NERC). The NERC was responsible for co-ordinating and overseeing international and national actors involved in the response. In the NERC, women's affairs were subsumed under the Psychosocial and Children's Affairs Pillar, led by the Ministry of Social Welfare, Gender and Children's Affairs and UNICEF. The 'Multi-sector Assessment of Gendered Impact of Ebola Virus Disease' survey noted that no specific meeting had been convened that focused on the needs of women and girls in the Ebola response (UN Women *et al.* 2014, 21, 26).

Oxfam's Rapid Gender Assessment in Sierra Leone showed that 70 per cent of national and district-level decision-makers in the Ebola response were male. When asked, all 25 'high-level' male policymakers argued against having a stand-alone gender plan in the Ebola response (Dietrich 2015). In comparison, a smaller group of 11 female 'highlevel' decision-makers within the Ebola response all argued for the need to have targeted actions to address women's particular needs (*ibid.*).

The importance of context-specific gender analysis

Getting policymakers to recognise gender as a factor that produces vulnerability can be a struggle; in order to be heard, practitioners make the case that women are disproportionately affected by crisis. As a result, staff and communities may receive the message that gender mainstreaming only responds to women's needs, overlooking the struggles facing men and boys in crisis-affected settings.

The Ebola response highlighted the ways in which rigorous research and gender analysis can inform better evidence-based policy and programming. A thorough gender analysis reveals the ways in which gender plays out in highly context-specific ways, requiring an approach tailored to the needs and interests of affected and at-risk communities.

For example, research showed that the social expectation that families would care for their loved ones during life and observe cultural practices of care for bodies after death created undeniable risks for those involved in overseeing and delivering care, particularly for women. A 'good' mother or wife was seen as one who cared for and provided for the sick, however, in Ebola she was explicitly told not to provide care and, in fact, told that providing care for the sick and deceased increased risk to the outbreak and its spread. This was because they are more likely to come into contact with bodily fluids or blood which is the primary method of transmission. In Sierra

Leone, bylaws were passed to ensure people did not behave in ways that would increase the spread of disease, installing fines for those who transgressed, however providing little option beyond reporting any suspected case (Ministry of Local Government and Rural Development, Sierra Leone 2014). These bylaws made illegal the homecare for or burial of anyone who was suspected of having Ebola.

Women were therefore put in a very difficult position. They risked either not fulfilling their duties as caregivers, causing significant distress to them and their family members, or risked spreading the disease if they did fulfil their role as a 'good' caregiver (wife/mother), which involved flouting the bylaws. In either case, they were exposed to stigma, and accusations of failure to fulfil expected duties.

A gender analysis that concluded with these observations might lead practitioners to assume from the outset that women will be more vulnerable to Ebola infection and, early in the crisis, data appeared to confirm that women were disproportionately at risk of Ebola infection, due to their role as caregivers (UNDP 2015, 2).

However, later analysis challenged this conclusion. In fact, the cumulative national data in Sierra Leone showed that infection rates among women were only slightly higher than those of men. In February 2015, out of a total of 11,132 confirmed and probable Ebola Virus Disease cases, 5,396 (48.4 per cent) were male, while 5,736 (51.6 per cent) were female (WHO 2015). Subsequent data also showed that, once infected, men faced a higher mortality rate than women (WHO Ebola Response Team 2016).

However, the relative parity of male and female infection rates could not be taken to mean that gender was not a relevant factor. Rather, rigorous gender analysis showed that the gendered division of labour in Sierra Leone put men and women at risk of Ebola infection in different ways. Although women faced high risks as household caregivers, men faced their own risks of infection due to their roles in transporting the sick. In several cases, the exposure of male motorcycle taxi drivers resulted in new chains of Ebola transmission in previously unexposed villages. An analysis that only considered women's vulnerability, or one that did not consider gender at all, risked overlooking these critical causal pathways, resulting in a response incapable of preventing further transmission of the virus.

Gender mainstreaming in WASH has made great strides in shedding light on previously neglected social issues, including women's roles and the gendered power relations that often harm women. However, the Ebola response highlighted the long-overdue need to move beyond an understanding of gender as relating only to women's vulnerability. Lessons learned from the Ebola outbreak should challenge the burden of proof that falls on gender mainstreaming practitioners to demonstrate that women are disproportionately diseased or dying before their concerns can be heard.

In the next section we focus in detail on how Oxfam could have improved our own WASH-Ebola response.

What could we have done better?

While Oxfam's WASH interventions created new spaces and structures within communities, such as CHVs which enabled gender parity, we could have done better to ensure an atmosphere to counterbalance structural gendered power inequalities

Our field visits confirmed what has been raised in other research reports, namely that gendered expectations of behaviour limited women's meaningful participation and comprehensive inclusion in the response. In Sierra Leone, CHVs stated that women are expected to stay at home; in community meetings, they sit behind the men and might be 'chased away' if male relatives object to their presence. A women's group complained that men exclude them from decision-making and do not inform them about meetings and trainings, particularly if the meeting involves stipend or *per diem* payments. A council woman noted that, historically, women were not supposed to speak in front of men, and could not act as chiefs or council members and their capacity to participate in community decision-making is greatly dependent on the influence of local female leaders and the attitudes of community chiefs (Minor and Kanneh 2015). During a workshop with CHVs in Sierra Leone, female team members reported that, even in the context of a workshop for Oxfam staff, women will censor themselves in the presence of men, limiting the contributions they could make when compared to female-only sessions.

Women's limited participation at household, community, regional, and national levels constrained their inclusion throughout the response, and Oxfam's WASH interventions did not go beyond the minimum standards

We could have done better in involving women in key Hygiene Promotion[2] approaches, even though women were targeted as beneficiaries. Ideally, we could have done more to consider women's access to information. Women were not included in the same circles, groups, and meetings where information was shared. In Liberia, our study (Minor 2014) revealed significant disparities in men's and women's access to Ebola prevention and treatment information in rural areas. A meeting with male leaders in Liberia demonstrated that men had a firm grasp on Ebola prevention and treatment messages. A concurrent focus group discussion with women found them brimming with questions, misinformation, and apprehensions. In Sierra Leone, women's focus group discussions with CHVs reported the same, highlighting that women were expected to protect their families but were unable to access the information required to do so (Carter *et al.* 2017a). Women reported that messages and information were passed down from traditional and community leaders who were men. Interviews with women in Sierra Leone reported that NGOs would enter their village and hold a meeting first with male leaders, who would in turn inform the others. Women were often not engaged directly in the first round of information dissemination. UN Women's report in Liberia also stated that educational levels correlated strongly with knowledge about Ebola; hence males were more likely to have heard about Ebola Treatment Centres than females (Korkoyah and Wreh 2015).

Ebola messaging targeted women primarily as mothers, and stressed fear-based approaches, failing to identify positive forms of engagement

Ebola campaigns placed great emphasis on targeting women and their traditional role as caregivers to stop the spread of Ebola. Messages were originally based in fear; highlighting the risk of death if women did not take measures to prevent infection or to seek help. The campaigns forbade women from caring for the sick – a critical part of their expected role as a 'good mother' – but did not provide them with alternatives. In Sierra Leone, women explained that it was simply not feasible to act the way the campaigns were instructing them to; that failure to care for their sick child would have made them feel like – and be seen as – a bad mother. One CHV explained that mothers were not able to simply 'abandon' their children at a treatment centre (Carter *et al.* 2017b). The campaigns were not developed together with the contribution of women, who could have provided advice on messages and images to better support the adoption of safe behaviour. For example, international handwashing campaigns target women with images of a good mother, who protects her child from illness by washing her hands. Mothers contributed to the creation of more inclusive campaign designs, by removing brand names from soap images, and including images of mothers washing their hands with ash when they did not have soap. This campaign was more successful than those that scolded mothers who did not practise handwashing. Our campaigns likewise would have benefited from the early inclusion of women's feedback in the construction and dissemination of Hygiene Promotion messaging.

The focus on women as mothers trivialised and reduced their roles in the response

We failed to include many specific women's groups in our response, such as traditional healers, birth attendants, and secret societies. In the early months of the response, this may have been due to the limited numbers and capacity of actors actively engaged in the response. By the time the international response scaled up (including Oxfam in October 2014), the crisis had become so great, that we struggled to find time to map out existing groups with whom we should be working. Women's secret societies were banned from carrying out female genital cutting (FGC),[3] but no additional attempt to work with them was launched. We may have overlooked the critical roles of women leaders in secret societies and burials; the importance of traditional birth attendants in rural health care; and the role of women in caregiving in general. In particular, as the research in Liberia showed, the role of women as community-based informal health-care providers and their impact on health-seeking behaviours was not sufficiently considered and included in our programmes (Minor 2014).

Lessons for the future: gender mainstreaming in WASH in Ebola

There are many insights from this research and too little space to discuss all of them. In this chapter we will focus on some key issues already raised as challenges by staff.

Reaffirming the importance of gender analysis for effective WASH programming

One of these key insights is that rigorous gender analysis is needed, and works to support effective programming. This means being sure we do not second-guess any finding, but also that we analyse our findings knowing that gender power relations disadvantage and marginalise women in the vast majority – perhaps all – contexts. In the course of first phase, Ebola response comprehensive context analysis was of utmost importance for WASH staff to begin contacting and including those most vulnerable to infection in programme planning and implementation. It was also essential to enable us to contribute to humanitarian programming messaging to contain the outbreak.

The deployment of an interdisciplinary research capacity to support national and international WASH teams in the field served as a constructive influencer in the WASH-Ebola programmes' development and for individual team members. The additional support helped WASH teams to move beyond only collecting sex and age disaggregated data, to a full gender analysis. Information and insights with importance for programme design were subsequently disseminated. While rapid gender analysis is of crucial importance, good data and good analysis are needed for good interventions. Often we expect programme teams to be able to run such analyses, however, given the time required on the response itself, this is rarely feasible. The survey revealed that the team of expert researchers working on the Ebola crisis were seen by WASH staff as their prime source of information on gendered power dynamics within the Ebola response.

Ensuring we learn from existing development programming

Rapid gender analysis is made easier and stronger if we integrate learning from development programmes around women's political participation and women's rights programming, when parachuting in and when handing-over in an emergency response.

Prior to the Ebola outbreak, both Sierra Leone and Liberia had ongoing programmes which focused on increasing women's participation, empowerment, and equality. These experiences were relevant to inform Community Outreach and WASH interventions: in particular, they offered information on existing social norms and gender roles. For example, one insight concerned women's leadership in Sierra Leone's Western Area where one council woman stated that, due to previous Oxfam programmes focused on increasing women's political participation, respect for women's leadership had grown significantly over the past ten years (Minor and Kanneh 2015).

Gaining a clear understanding of existing development programmes should be part of the WASH teams' rapid scale-up. While humanitarian teams often report on doing this, or recommend it for future, it remains challenging. Having a support team (such as the gender advisors, epidemiologists, and anthropologists) in addition to the rapid response WASH team to provide a more in-depth context analysis would further facilitate information translation between the two programmes. This is important for us to seize opportunities in terms of ensuring continuities for women's participation, regardless of the context and response at the time.

Ensuring women's full and equal participation in leadership

The need to include women fully and equally in programme design and implementation is separate from the last point. Indeed, women's greater participation at these levels may have improved the analysis by encouraging not only a focus on women as unpaid carers, but a focus on men's roles as transport drivers, revealing the complexity of how Ebola was affecting, and affected by, gender roles and relations.

In development and humanitarian work generally, women still face barriers to their participation and leadership and, as described earlier, this was particularly seen by staff as a problem in the rapid, large-scale, and militarised national-level Ebola response. Within Oxfam's own response, participation of women is also seen as an issue and Oxfam WASH teams have incorporated minimum checklists for equal and equitable access into their daily practice. Our research and experience suggests WASH staff in Oxfam's Ebola response naturally expected gender parity within Oxfam teams. They aspired to this in their work with CHVs, and the idea that women and men receive the same training and payments for their work are quite standard by now.

In our view, the Ebola experience shows the need to be bold in assuming women are politically under-represented, and faster and more creative in addressing this prevailing pattern, to allow for meaningful participation. We do not have to wait for gender analysis to evidence women's under-representation in high-level decision-making spaces. Militarised contexts, top-down decision-making structures, and sidelining of community health structures should be a good indication that women are likely to be sidelined from providing and receiving information, participating, and decision-making.

In consequence, humanitarian WASH teams need to be faster to acknowledge this shortage of women in leadership of crises and address it. They can do so using locally appropriate means, creating women-only spaces, helping to raise women's opinion and voices, engaging with women's organisations, serving as transmitters of women's opinions, and ensuring they create spaces to invite women to use to raise their issues and be heard on their own. It is not only about presence, but about meaningful participation, and proactively reaching out. As such, community engagement and WASH programmes should seek to bridge the gap between the high-level decision-makers, (male) community leaders, and women, providing targeted information and communication opportunities for women.

Working with women in their community roles

In the Ebola response, Oxfam's WASH teams were fast to understand women's important role as primary caregivers and to target mothers in the programme, as highlighted earlier. Effective WASH programming in the Ebola context required a properly gendered response that moved beyond stereotypes and narrow understandings of gender mainstreaming as being concerned with women only.

We have argued that WASH practitioners also need to be open to moving beyond a focus on women's unpaid care work. Programming effectively often involves considering women's roles in the paid economy, but it could also involve recognising other unpaid community work they undertake. This often, but not always, focuses on health. Anthropological research (Minor 2014) identified the important role of women as communitybased health-care providers in Liberia, which we had previously failed to include. The study found that women, as primary caregivers, are the ones who know whether a relative or neighbour is sick, and circulate that knowledge among other women.

Engaging with local women's groups would create a system of community accountability for the referral and treatment of people who fall ill. Traditional Trained Midwives in particular tend to provide a locus of shared confidentiality among women, and often make up a critical part of rural health systems (*ibid.*). Similarly, in Sierra Leone, working with traditional birth attendants and female traditional healers to engage in discussions on safe sexual and reproductive health practices, safe burial, and access information and communication networks among women needs to be part of the first-phase response.

The need to work with unlikely partners when the need arises

This takes us to the next point: the need to focus on the importance of delivering a highquality crisis response may require working with women who are not supporting the empowerment of women and gender equality goals: or at least, to consider doing so.

In Ebola, our inability to engage with female secret societies and traditional doctors who practised FGC eliminated a portal to engage with women. It is easy to only work with partners and groups who have the same ways of thinking or similar mandates to our own, however, what do we do when this negates large groups of the population?

The research from the Ebola response demonstrates that in a crisis, we may need to dialogue and partner with groups who will ensure our access in the best and most appropriate way to vulnerable groups, regardless of their mandate. Female elders who were secret society members and leaders were critical in burial practices as the ones to wash and take care of bodies. Engaging with them at that level may perhaps lead to progressive longer-term change in the future. By ignoring these groups, we have essentially said we will only work with like-minded people and therefore eliminate opportunities for behaviour change by not engaging with those who behave differently.

Ensuring effective health messaging and campaigns using a gender perspective

The research showed that gender mainstreaming into Ebola response needed to involve considering appropriate ways to deliver health messaging to women and girls, and to traditionally marginalised groups. In the context of the top-down Ebola response, messaging had to follow co-ordination and sign-off, and means of dissemination included billboards, radio, and other formal means. Informal messaging was clearly important also.

In crises like Ebola, there is a need to move in future from standardised messages that fail to provide information and alternative practice options in ways that are meaningful to women. The information provided, language, and imagery needed not only to inform communities, but also to address barriers that stop someone from acting on the messages. Including women in the design of the campaigns can ensure that a greater number of people are reached.

Oxfam's Ebola response aimed to fill information gaps on health messaging quickly. We relied on existing social dynamics via CHVs and community leaders. However, our research shows this was not adequate, as women did not have the same access to information as men.

Communication should be two-way, with women's requests taken seriously, either ensuring better messaging or providing access to requests, as examples around protective gear showed. Although the messages were clear regarding care for the sick, given the initial very limited availability and access to treatment facilities, providing protective gear to communities (women) may be an option that would still allow women to provide care in a safe manner. While this could be argued as encouraging high-risk behaviour, studies have shown that high-risk practices continued late into the response and this may provide a quick option in early phases to encourage treatment-seeking rather than push further high-risk practices that go unreported.

Conclusion

The positive spirit of the survey we embarked on for this chapter was that WASH professionals involved in Oxfam's Ebola response acknowledged that 'gender work' is more than a box-ticking exercise and about more than female headcount, a focus on women only, or even a focus on caring work in the household. In addition, gender mainstreaming has the potential to do more than ensure access to facilities to women. As survey respondents stated, gender mainstreaming in Ebola provided them with the space to ask critical questions about context, including being able to identify gaps in participation of women's secret societies and traditional healers, and shape our programmes to be more inclusive, building a better dialogue with communities. In consequence, gender mainstreaming is an asset with the potential to improve humanitarian interventions in terms of analysis by aiding understanding of the underlying power dynamics and cultural context.

Gender mainstreaming is not a one-off exercise, but recurrent, and it requires critical thinking as situations also change. No generic checklist can tell you how to do it in a specific context – changes across countries (Sierra Leone and Liberia), across urban–rural divide, across different communities, religions, and social practices. The vast body of knowledge, guidelines, and checklists that has led to the adoption of minimum standards on gender in WASH practice, covered the basics on equal and equitable access of women and girls. However, in cases of complex emergency such as Ebola, WASH practitioners needed to be faster, being bolder, more creative, and more critical, in order to achieve the highest quality programme. It is not about doing new things, it is about doing the things we already do in a better and more reflective way.

Notes

1. Ebola Treatment Units (ETU) were used in Liberia as treatment units for Ebola patients (Washington and Meltzer 2015). In Sierra Leone, comparable structures were used called Ebola Treatment Centres (ETC) (Gulland 2014). The ETUs and ETCs were set up with the same structures and treatment approaches, only with different names.
2. Hygiene Promotion approaches in Ebola consisted of working with CHVs and Oxfam staff to conduct house-to-house visits, small group discussions (as large gatherings were not permitted), and radio messages which provided communities with information on prevention, detection, and control (first response) to Ebola, while promoting treatment-seeking and creating a space to answer questions regarding Ebola.
3. FGC (also known as female genital mutilation – FGM) in Sierra Leone is an act performed as part of the initiation ceremony into the Bondo Society. This society is a traditional, secret women's society, and it is from FGM performed by the Bondo Society that girls (ages 15–19 years) are then recognised as women within their communities (Bjälkander *et al.* 2016, e447).

Notes on contributors

Simone E. Carter is Head of the social sciences analysis cell for Unicef in DRC ebola response. Email: simoneelysecarter@gmail.com

Luisa Maria Dietrich is a Gender Justice Specialist. Email: Luisa. Dietrich@gmail.com

Olive Melissa Minor is a Research and Evaluation Specialist. Email: olive.m.minor@gmail.com

ORCID

Simone E. Carter http://orcid.org/0000-0003-3818-3538
Luisa Maria Dietrich http://orcid.org/0000-0003-4816-8016
Olive Melissa Minor http://orcid.org/0000-0002-1460-6236

References

Bjälkander, Owolabi, Helena Nordenstedt, Kim Brolin and Anna Mia Ekström (2016) 'FGM in the time of Ebola—carpe opportunitatem', *The Lancet Global Health* 4(7): e447–e448 (last checked 24 May 2017)

Carter, Simone, Marion O'Reilly, Vivien Walden, Jack Frith-Powell, Alpha Umar Kargbo and Eva Niederberger (2017a) 'Barriers and enablers to treatment-seeking behavior and causes of high-risk practices in Ebola: a case study from Sierra Leone', *The Journal of Health Communication*, (in press)

Carter, Simone Carter, Marion O'Reilly, Jack Frith-Powell, Alpha Umar Kargbo, Daniel Byrne and Eva Niederberger (2017b) 'Treatment-seeking and Ebola community care centers in Sierra Leone: a qualitative study', *The Journal of Health Communication*, (in press)

CDC (2014) Data available at https://www.cdc.gov/vhf/ebola/out-breaks/2014-west-africa (last checked 23 May 2017)

Clifton, Deborah (1999) *A Little Gender Handbook for Emergencies or Just Plain Common Sense*, Oxford: Oxfam GB

Dietrich, L. (2015) 'Oxfam gender brief for programming and advocacy: The impact of Ebola virus disease in Sierra Leone', Oxfam internal document

Gulland, Anne (2014) 'UK built Ebola treatment centre opens in Sierra Leone', *BMJ* 349: g6704, http://www.bmj.com/content/349/bmj.g6704 (last checked 24 May 2017)

Kloosterman, Jeanette (2014) *Transformative Leadership for Women's Rights: An Oxfam Guide*, Oxford: Oxfam International

Korkoyah, Jr., Dala T. and Francis F. Wreh (2015) *Ebola Impact Revealed: An Assessment of the Differing Impact of the Outbreak on Women and Men in Liberia*, UN Women, Oxfam, Ministry of Gender, Children and Social Protection, https://www.oxfam.org/sites/www.oxfam.org/files/file_attachments/rr-ebola-impact-women-men-liberia-010715-en.pdf (last checked 24 May 2017)

Médecins Sans Frontières (2014) 'MSF calls outbreak out of control on June 23 2014', http://www.doctorswithoutborders.org/news-stories/press-release/ebola-massive-deployment-needed-fight-epidemic-west-africa (last checked 24 May 2017)

Médecins Sans Frontières (2015) *Pushed to the Limit and Beyond: A year into the largest ever Ebola outbreak*. Report, MSF, https://www.doctorswithout borders.org/sites/usa/files/msf143061.pdf (last checked 24 May 2017)

Ministry of Local Government and Rural Development, Sierra Leone (2014) *By-Laws for All Chiefdoms in Sierra Leone Formulated by the National Council of Paramount Chiefs and Ministry of Local Government and Rural Development*

Geared Towards the Prevention of Ebola and Other Diseases, available at https://www.humanitarianresponse.info/system/files/documents/files/by-laws.pdf (last checked 24 May 2017)

Minor, Olive Melissa (2014) *Community perceptions of Ebola Response Efforts in Liberia: Montserrado and Nimba Counties*, http://www.ebola-anthropology.net/wp-content/uploads/2015/02/OxfamMMinorPeters-Liberia-Anthro-report_Dec2014.pdf (last checked 24 May 2017)

Minor, Olive Melissa and Sheku Sharix Kanneh (2015) *Ebola and Accusation: Gender Dimensions of Stigma in Sierra Leone's Ebola Response*, https://www.researchgate.net/publication/308048410_Ebola_and_Accusation_Gender_Dimensions_of_Stigma_in_Sierra_Leone's_Ebola_Response (last checked 6 June 2017)

Oxfam (2012) *Ending Violence against Women: An Oxfam Guide*, Oxford: Oxfam International, https://www.oxfam.org/sites/www.oxfam.org/files/ending-violence-against-women-oxfam-guide-nov2012.pdf (last checked 24 May 2017)

Oxfam (2013) *Oxfam Minimum Standards for Gender in Emergencies*, Oxford: Oxford International, https://www.oxfam.org/en/research/minimum-standards-gender-emergencies (last checked 24 May 2017)

Oxfam (2017) *Gender Leadership in Humanitarian Action: Institutionalizing Gender in Emergencies – Bridging Policy and Practice in the Humanitarian System*, Oxford: Oxfam, http://policy-practice.oxfam.org.uk/publications/training-manual-gender-leadership-in-humanitarian-action-620215 (last checked 24 May 2017)

Taqi, Fatmatta (2015) 'Rapid gender assessment report of the Ebola response on OXFAM Sierra Leone's Operational Areas', Oxfam Sierra Leone internal document

UNDP (2015) 'UNDP Africa policy brief note: confronting the gender impact of Ebola virus disease in Guinea, Liberia, and Sierra Leone', 2(1), available at http://reliefweb.int/sites/reliefweb.int/files/resources/RBA%20Policy%20Note%20Vol%202%20No%201%202015_Gender.pdf (last checked 24 May 2017)

UN Women Ministry of Social Welfare, Gender and Children's Affairs, Statistics Sierra Leone and Oxfam (2014) 'Report of the multisector impact assessment of gender dimensions of the Ebola Virus Disease (EVD) December, available at https://awdf.org/wp-content/uploads/FINAL-REPORT-OFTHE-Multi-Sectoral-GENDER-Impact-Assessment_Launchedon_24th-Feb-2015_Family_kingdom_Resort.pdf (last checked 6 June 2017)

Washington, Michael L. and Martin L. Meltzer (2015) 'Effectiveness of Ebola treatment units and community care centers — Liberia', September 23–October 31, 2014, https://www.cdc.gov/mmwr/preview/mmwrhtml/mm6403a6.htm (last checked 24 May 2017)

WHO (2015) 'Ebola situation report', 25 February, http://apps.who.int/ebola/en/ebola-situation-report/situation-reports/ebola-situation-report-25-february-2015 (last checked 24 May 2017)

WHO Ebola Response Team (2016) 'Ebola virus disease among male and female persons in West Africa', *New England Journal of Medicine* 374: 96–98, http://www.nejm.org/doi/full/10.1056/NEJMc1510305#t=chapter (last checked 24 May 2017), DOI: 10.1056/NEJMc1510305

CHAPTER 5

Women's environmental health activism around waste and plastic pollution in the coastal wetlands of Yucatán

Anne-Marie Hanson

Abstract

This chapter focuses on women's grassroots organisations and their role in confronting waste-induced water, health, and development challenges in low-lying tropical coastal areas. As a case study, the chapter will focus on women's waste management and plastics recycling organisations in Yucatán, Mexico and their role in preventing water-borne diseases and educating the community on the links between garbage and human health. Women educate the community on the links between garbage and human health; challenge exclusionary gender norms by increasing women's participation in community sustainable development, and improve urban conditions in the coastal wetlands. I draw from over 400 surveys with coastal residents and 14 oral histories with coastal women, to underscore the muddy links that connect sanitation to gendered responsibility and the exclusionary spaces of urban development and ecological restoration in the swamps. The information shared through the histories and broad surveys emphasises how gendered roles and expectations are critical variables in shaping social difference, ecological degradation, and human health in low-lying coastal areas and cities.

Keywords: Recycling; waste; women's grassroots organisations; coastal wetlands; Yucatán; México

Introduction

Coastal Yucatán, Mexico, is often portrayed as an eco-tourist paradise filled with internationally protected corridors of wetlands, marine life, coastal dunes, and tens of thousands of pink flamingoes. This pristine image, however, muddles the reality of many coastal residents who face challenges to health and development due to the increasing presence of non-organic wastes and plastic pollution in coastal wetlands, estuaries, and freshwater aquifers. Inflows of garbage from tourism, rapid urbanisation, and changing consumption patterns pose serious threats to the region, such as: reduced standards of living for coastal

http://dx.doi.org/10.3362/9781788530866.005

residents, increased illness related to waste decomposition in flood zones, damage to protected wetlands and marine ecosystems, and threats to the region's image as a desirable eco-tourist destination (Cob Chay 2011; Lliteras 2009).

Internationally, the overflow of land-based plastic wastes into the oceans is one of the most pervasive pollution problems faced by the Earth today (UNEP 2016). Over 20 million tons of plastic are estimated to reach the oceans each year. Plastics are now ubiquitous to the ocean, found in every ocean and on coastlines from the Arctic through the tropics to Antarctica. Single-use disposable food containers and packaging, together with plastic bags, make up the largest components of marine and coastal plastic litter (UNEP 2016). In recent years, a large amount of research has been dedicated to understanding the harmful effects of plastic pollution on marine species and ecosystems.[1] Marine plastic pollution has impacted several animal species worldwide, including the majority of all sea turtle species, and almost half of all seabird species and marine mammal species (Bergmann *et al.* 2015; UNEP 2016).

Most studies focused on social behaviours related to plastic waste and informal waste management, however, have focused on large, and often inland, urban centres. Still, almost half of the world's population now live within 150 km of a coastline, and by 2025 that figure is likely to double to over 6 billion (UN-OCEANS 2013). In many parts of the world, women and poor communities take on the responsibility of waste reduction and plastics recycling due to disorganised or absent state support for urban and coastal waste issues (Beall 2006). The lack of support for waste services or waste workers in many politically marginalised areas has also led diverse grassroots community groups to organise together in order to seek environmental justice, political representation for environmental health concerns, economic opportunities, and overall community well-being.[2]

In this chapter, I focus on two women's grassroots organisations in Yucatán, and their role in confronting waste-induced water, health, and development challenges in low-lying tropical coastal areas. Their work demonstrates the social norms and gendered responsibilities associated with disposal and removal of the increasing amounts of house-hold, tourist, and marine plastic debris found in residential and public coastal areas. This chapter also demonstrates the waste management responsibilities assumed by grassroots women's organisations, and positions these groups as primary drivers of gendered social change and urban sustainability in a region characterised for its rural activities in conserving tropical coastal landscapes. In particular, I will address women's waste management and plastics recycling organisations in Yucatán, Mexico and their role in (1) preventing diseases caused by garbage decomposition in the wetlands, (2) challenging exclusionary gender norms by increasing women's participation in community sustainable development, and (3) improving urban conditions in the coastal wetlands.

The chapter begins by discussing the gendered context of conservation space, tourism, and urbanisation in coastal Yucatán. I then provide a section on the history of the women's groups, before presenting my ethnographic evidence and analysis. The research that informs this chapter is based on ethnographic fieldwork conducted in Yucatán between 2009 and 2014.

Although I collected data in a variety of formats, for this paper, the focus is primarily on oral histories, surveys, and participant observation through garbage activities. Participant observation in this case included my participation in collection of plastic bottles and recyclables with the women's group, Chen Kole 'Lob (*sic*) (meaning 'only women' in Yucatec Maya), as well as informal conversations and various kinds of formal and informal interviews. I attended monthly meetings of the inter-municipal composting group, Las Costeras ('coastal women' in Spanish), and participated by helping out with the different steps of seaweed collection and composting. Through participant observation, I was able to engage in women's daily activities and better understand the everyday practices and perspectives of residents in Celestún. More importantly, this enabled me to understand the perspectives of women who choose to collect garbage and recyclable materials.

I also draw from over 400 surveys with coastal residents and 14 oral histories with coastal women to underscore the muddy links that connect sanitation to gendered responsibility and the exclusionary spaces of urban development and ecological restoration in the swamps. The information shared through the histories and broad surveys emphasises how gendered roles and expectations are critical variables in shaping social difference, ecological degradation, and human health in low-lying coastal areas and cities.

Gendered spaces of conservation and urban development in coastal Yucatán

Conservation

The coast of Yucatán is home to several types of biodiverse coastal and marine ecosystems, including mangrove swamps and wetlands that have played an important part in the local economy for thousands of years (Batllori-Sampedro *et al.* 1999). Regional vegetation includes a mixture of coastal dunes, mangroves, *petenes* (tropical plant colonies surrounding cenotes or freshwater springs), flooded wetlands, lowland jungle, and tropical dry forest (Acosta-Lugo *et al.* 2010). These ecosystems are refuge for many endemic and migratory species, they support commercial and recreational fisheries, are major tourist attractions, and are home to several thousand coastal residents. Erosion of the coast is a serious contemporary problem that may be a result of climate change as well as unsustainable tourism development and rapid urbanisation along the coast.

In working to protect the region's wetlands and biodiverse coastal habitats, environmental protection efforts have received much national and international attention since the 1980s, but particularly in the last 30 years with programmes funded by the World Bank, Global Environment Fund, and the Mesoamerican Biological Corridor (García de Fuentes *et al.* 2011). There are currently five protected conservation areas, including two federal biosphere reserves and three state reserves.

State and internationally funded sustainable development programmes often encourage livelihood shifts that promote conservation, and in doing so, often focus on biodiversity protection activities as means towards economic development. The development of tourism activities, in particular, is tightly linked with conservation areas and interests in the region (García de Fuentes and Xool 2012). Many development programmes are specifically focused on seasonal, resource-dependent activities, like sustainable fishing and eco-tourism in or near conservation areas. These attempts to protect nature by fixing livelihood activities in time (fishing and tourism seasons) and space (within protected corridors) have led to conflicts among coastal residents, as social inequalities also become 'fixed', through embodied environmental practices and their uneven expectations for urban or rural behaviours in small coastal cities.

Urbanisation and local tourism development

In northwestern Yucatán, there are 13 small, but growing urban areas located within or adjacent to protected conservation spaces (Hanson 2016). Although most are small by global urban standards (that is, many of the municipalities have more than 2,500 but less than 15,000 people) (INEGI 2015), the coastal towns in Yucatán nearly quadrupled in population between 1970 and 2000 (Batllori-Sampedro *et al.* 2006). These towns have also undergone multiple political and spatial (territorial) reorganisations in the last several decades, and coastal residents are continuously responding to changes in national and international regulations for industry, conservation, and tourism (Fraga 2006; Doyon 2008). A majority of residents in the region migrated there from the interior of the peninsula following the collapse of the henequen (a type of fibre) export industry. Due to an agricultural-economic crisis in the interior of the state, in the 1980s, state economic development programmes (e.g. El Programa de Reordenamiento Henequenero y Desarrollo Integral de Yucatán) gave financial credits to farmers to move to coastal areas and participate in the then growing export fishing industry (Baños Ramírez 2003). Since that time, people have continued to migrate to the coastal cities from the interior of the state and from drought or flood-stricken areas of the Peninsula (e.g. Tabasco and central Yucatán state).

Even with their relatively small size, most people living in coastal Yucatán consider that they live in urban areas (from surveys), and their consumption activities are similar to those in large cities. And yet, nearly all of the economic activities prevalent in Celestún are seasonal and are heavily dependent on natural resources and government financial support. Apart from fishing, other economic activities include artisanal salt extraction, tourism (hotel/restaurant), eco-tourism, and a small number of artisan and aquaculture co-operatives. Following the international recognition of Yucatán's Biosphere Reserves in 2004, the region has received a steady increase in the number of tourists.

Eco-tourism has been heavily promoted, and there are several small eco-tourism co-operatives (38 or more according to García de Fuentes and Xool Koh 2012, 174) that offer tours to see flamingoes, and to participate in hiking, biking, kayak, birding tours, seasonal duck hunting, among other activities in or near the region's conservation areas.

Most sustainable development policies in Mexico stress the need for more participation from both men and women in the protection of the nation's natural heritage.[3] In fact, participation in Mexican environmental policy is in reality no longer a question, but an imperative. Enhanced participation of women and communities in resource management is central to project design, but there is not always clear evidence of how such programmes benefit local women or communities (Harris 2009). While some programmes solicit gender-mainstreaming efforts, government work subsidies in and near natural protected areas in Yucatán tend to provide incentives to participate in eco-tourism or join co-operatives for sustainable fishing – two male-dominated activities. Women participate in these activities, but are not often direct recipients of work-related subsidies. Women and children participate by filleting fish, extracting pulp from crabs, or processing fish for different types of exported fish products. These activities are most frequently done in individual homes.

At one point, over 300 families in the town of Celestún alone participated in these activities, but currently fewer than 100 women fillet fish for the INPESMAR fish freezer and they are paid ten pesos per kilogram of fillets. To fillet 15–30 kilos of fish takes about four to eight hours of work, and earns about 70–140 pesos (US$6–12). Fish processing declined with the increase in people living in the region, which led to fewer fish available and more federal regulations regarding when and how many of each fish species can be caught in any season (interviews, 2011).

Furthermore, state and international sustainable development projects in this region have largely prioritised the protection of wetlands from unsanitary human activities, rather than directly addressing the human and environmental health issues surrounding urban sprawl in the wetlands, such as sanitation and waste and wastewater management. Few development interventions have focused on the social and material problems linked to daily urban practices in the growing coastal towns. Everyday consumption, waste, and sanitation issues in urban areas have been under-prioritised at many levels of government unless they are framed as threats to coastal ecosystems and conservation. Instead, in many small coastal cities, women have assumed many of the responsibilities for improving urban conditions and preventing water-borne diseases through community-based organised waste management and education activities.

Garbage in the wetlands

In Yucatán, garbage governance is entangled in gendered networks of knowledge, practice, and politics, and is linked to questions of environmental responsibility and informal urban development. The garbage problem in coastal Yucatán is also the result of the gradual merging of social, political, and environmental networks that historically were – and for the most part continue to be – managed in separate urban or rural policy spheres.

The complexity of geographic, economic, political, and social aspects is part of a nation-wide waste problem. Most environmental policies in Mexico do not directly support recovery activities nor stimulate growth of the recycling industry. This has often hindered government reforms (at all scales) towards more efficient collection, recovery, and recycling systems and new waste management technologies (Schwanse 2011). For example, in the last 30 years, individual consumption of plastic products was heavily promoted throughout Mexico. This consumption has dramatically increased in both rural and urban areas. Furthermore, although most coastal communities are still very small by global urban standards, consumption habits are similar to large cities. The convenience of single-use plastics, the lack of clean drinking water, and easy access to comida *chatarra* (junk food) have led to excessive numbers of single-use plastic bags, beverage bottles, and food packaging as common, everyday waste items.

Based on recent estimates, the small cities of coastal Yucatán continue to have some of the least organised garbage collection programmes in the state, where in some areas less than 6 per cent of garbage is deposited in controlled sites (SEDUMA 2009). While most restaurants and hotels have regular garbage collection (approximately 84 per cent), a much smaller percentage of residential areas have regular garbage collection (14 per cent for informal residences, and up to 65 per cent for formal residences) (Vásquez Avila *et al.* 2011, 56). Instead, some garbage is burned, and much is used for filling in terrains in order to expand and stabilise yards located in annual flood zones. Recycling behaviours are welcome and promoted by government agencies and some local authorities, but there are few resources allocated for services and products for this sector (Schwanse 2011). In the case of many small coastal towns, municipal governments have only enough funds to fund a mayor and basic services partially.

Also, the coastal population quadrupled in size without sufficient funds or infrastructure for urban services like drainage, sewage disposal, or garbage collection. The lack of services is largely attributed to this rapid growth and lack of consistent urban planning. While electricity is accessible to most residential areas (94 per cent), only 74 per cent of homes have drainage, and 15 or more per cent of homes are without toilets or piped water (INEGI 2015, 113–4).

Recent urbanisation in northwestern Yucatán occurred primarily in the region's wetlands, where pervious soils were partially stabilised to accommodate rapid growth. Historically, non-organic wastes such as plastic bottles, scrap metal, and derelict construction materials have been use as inexpensive stabilising materials to fill in uneven or eroding backyards. Today, as a result, many homes in coastal towns are located on the edges of wetlands or lagoons that have doubled as open-air dumps due to lack of alternate disposal sites or in areas where individuals used municipal solid wastes to fill in unstable land.

This unplanned urbanisation interrupts natural flows of fresh water, disrupts and pollutes ecosystems, and also puts residents at higher risks from climate change-induced weather patterns and annual flooding. The combination of solid wastes and lack of drainage in many informal residential areas has also been linked to the proliferation of infectious disease vectors – in particular mosquitoes and bacteria. Coastal communities also associate this waste decomposition to past outbreaks of cholera, dengue, and rotavirus.

Above all other urban features, garbage is a particular problem that is now well noted in regional newspapers as a threat to conservation of wetlands and to the local tourism and fishing industries. Newspaper chapters describe garbage as an indicator of social backwardness and a threat to health and tourism (Lliteras 2009). One chapter described several coastal towns as a disgrace to the coastal landscape, stuck in a rut of poverty and squalor, and in urgent need of improved urban services (Cob Chay and Ucán Chan 2010). Coastal researcher Robles de Benito also notes in a study on community social relations with the biosphere reserve that the presence of garbage in Celestún and other coastal communities, 'deteriorates the quality of the landscape, and negatively affects the quality of life of residents, as well as the image for tourism' (Robles de Benito 2005, 64).

Fifteen per cent of coastal residents view the region's garbage problems as the responsibility of individual households, and this view was especially prevalent for residents with homes in stable lands and where the garbage collection trucks regularly pass. However, the majority of residents interviewed (80 per cent) consider the garbage problem to be primarily the responsibility of the municipal government, who they also consider to be uninterested in the topic as it relates to residential areas. A number of residents view the lack of written plans for garbage and other urban services in residential areas as typical examples of government disinterest and corruption (interviews, April and June 2011). This was especially true for those residents who live on edges of the *cienaga* (lagoon) and smaller ponds. As one resident with a house on the *cienaga* explained:

> The [municipal] government doesn't really care about garbage. We have lived this way for a long time. I would like to move my house, but there is nowhere to build that I can afford, so we stay. We never had a garbage truck pass here; it won't come because the roads are too bad. Now we recycle bottles, but that is for money. We used to throw them behind the house. The municipio is fixing the roads to private hotels. We can't even go there, but that's what they fix first. Millions of pesos to fix those roads, because they are for the wealthy tourists. (Interview, Celestún, June 2011)

As another coastal resident and hotel owner in northern Yucatán asserted:

> Ha! You're going to study garbage in Yucatán? Well, that's easy. There's a lot of garbage and very little interest in it. Nobody cares about garbage here. It's that most people here don't have anything, so why are

they going to care about garbage? ... When your house is made of cardboard and you shit in the swamps, garbage is the least of your concerns. (Interview with hotel owner, February 2011)

The waste problem, however, is not due to household consumption alone. The small towns in the region receive millions of tourists each year. These tourists often arrive on the beach or wetlands tours with food containers and disposable items that they do not take with them when they return home. The amount of solid waste and plastic waste can increase 100 times the normal level during high tourist seasons. Increasingly, severe seasonal weather patterns, and the gradual rise in sea level, also produce more extreme and larger areas of annual flooding in these coastal cities, and intensified tropical storms erode beaches and wash ashore thousands of tons of marine litter (mainly plastics) each year (UNEP 2006).

Women's groups work to promote community health through garbage clean-up

The increasing amounts of non-organic garbage (e.g. plastic bottles, bags, and other containers) and lack of controlled final disposal are growing concerns for environmental health and public health. Garbage contaminates backyards, protected wetlands, and community freshwater sources. As coastal communities are built upon the unstable soils of the coastal wetlands, residents' homes are continuously confronted with annual flooding and hurricanes. The structural and health concerns associated with the overflow of garbage particularly interested local women, who have been addressing this issue for over 20 years. In small towns all along the coast of Yucatán, women are the main advocates for community waste management, forming grassroots recycling and composting groups, as well as inter-municipal garbage alliances.

For a long period of time, development scholars and practitioners viewed women as outside the central arena of economic development and primarily in need of health or other welfare assistance in their roles as mothers and housewives (Moser 1993). Separate roles for women in the management of resources are not always acknowledged. Often, 'women's activities have been considered "duties" and not "work," because they are not paid for doing them' (Rimarachín Cabrera *et al.* 2001, 86). In coastal Yucatán Peninsula, this view has been replicated. Although some international donors and state organisations have gender-related goals that specify inclusion of women as direct beneficiaries of projects, most conservation and development projects generally target men as fishermen and tourism operators.

Yet, rather than focus on women's organisations as related to their vulnerabilities and exclusion in seemingly participatory development and conservation processes, we found that women from (and despite) their marginalised position, are very active in the community efforts to mitigate negative effects of environmental change on natural resources (Hanson and Buechler 2015).

Following Katy Jenkins' study of women's grassroots health-care workers in Ecuador, our own study frames grassroots women organisers as 'dynamic, albeit under-valued, activists, rather than relying on more jaded images of grassroots women organizing simply for survival' (Jenkins 2008, 156). In coastal Yucatán, women did not regularly receive government subsidies for preferred activities in fishing and eco-tourism, but they created a venue for their participation and recognition in sustainable development through garbage management, motivated by concern for human health and the tourism industries in their communities.

Two women's grassroots organisations in Yucatán have played a large role in confronting waste-induced water, health, and development challenges in the area. Between 1997 and 2002, small groups of coastal women organised to collect plastic bottles and other recyclables, to gather and compost seaweed that washed up on beaches following tropical storms, and to organise wetlands and beach clean-up projects in their communities. Women, who were already largely in charge of household garbage, became interested in larger collective projects of community garbage management. Household and residential garbage management is largely seen as an issue of cleanliness and health, linked to women's domestic responsibilities. Surveys of households with both men and women living in the home indicate residents' view that women are primarily responsible for keeping houses and yards clean (93 per cent of respondents), for household recycling (63 per cent of respondents), and for disposing of organic and food wastes (84 per cent of respondents). Men are most often considered responsible for municipal street cleaning, since men are employed as street sweepers, and for collecting garbage in the city trucks (interviews, April 2011).

Las Costeras began as a group of 25 women who organised in 1997 in the town of Dzilam de Bravo, motivated by the need to protect their communities from the health issues linked to waste and seaweed decomposition on beaches, and to attract tourists. This was the first group to collect the washed-up seaweed in order to turn it into compost that is then later sold to local inland farmers or used in community gardens. Las Costeras has since grown to include over 400 women in several coastal towns.

In addition to Las Costeras, the recycling group Chen Kole 'Lob, meaning 'only women' in Yucatec Maya, began in 2002 with 17 women who collect plastic bottles and organise wetlands clean-up projects. They began to organise around the issues following a lecture given at a bi-monthly meeting of Oportunidades in 2002, a national development programme that gives small stipends to poor women with children who regularly attend school (interviews, March 2011).

Women were especially concerned with the overflow of garbage in providing breeding grounds for dengue-carrying mosquitos and the links between decaying wastes in the water stream and the cholera outbreaks that affected many coastal residents in the 1990s and early 2000s (interviews, April 2012). Women also organised yearly wetlands and beach clean-up projects that bring temporary work grants to hundreds of community members (both men and women). The women have been very proactive in seeking out funding efforts for these projects. Women view this work as an opportunity for better community health and to make small contributions to their families' economic situations.

Local expectations that women would not work long hours outside the home led to this rarely happening prior to the garbage clean-up. Because of this, and also a general lack of support and even stigmatisation of the idea of cleaning up garbage in small coastal cities, at times the women were criticised for their work with garbage (Hanson 2015). Recycling, composting, and wetland clean-up are also tasks that require complicated organising, and they involve very hard work with little financial gain. Many members of both women's groups explained that they were scrutinised or even belittled by other town residents, for being *pepenadoras* (scavengers), and for embarrassing themselves by collecting other people's waste bottles. Several women explained to me that they were often defending themselves and validating why they would bother cleaning the trash that washed up on beaches, or was left there as litter by other people or tourists.

One woman in particular defended her work by describing how garbage had value:

> You know, they have teased us plenty. They tell me 'you are dirty' and 'like to play with garbage' ... but as much as they tease us, they now see that it is not garbage, it is money thrown away. It is not much, but it is something. It is capital. (Interview, Sisal, November 2012)

Another woman told me they did the work because men are only interested in fishing and tourism, and women are better at keeping things clean:

> As women we are always cleaning anyway ... if we don't clean our yards, if we don't sweep, the winds or the water [from flooding] brings the garbage back into our houses. (Interview, Celestún, August 2012)

In many cases, husbands and male family members were initially unsupportive or even objected to women's participation in garbage work. As one women explained:

> There are a lot of 'delicate' husbands here [*Vemos que hay muchos esposos delicados aquí*]. They don't want us to work with garbage. They said we were strange, even stupid, dirty, they called us scavengers [*pepenadoras nos dijeron*]. (Interviews, April 2012)

As another women further asserted, the lack of municipal support for waste management and health concerns was enough to organise, despite initial backlash from some men and other community members:

> The thing is ... nobody recycled, it was just us. It was too much [garbage]. After several years we finally started seeing that people noticed what we were doing. They asked us 'what do you do with all those bottles?' Well, we sell them! At 20 cents a kilo. And everyone said, '*Ay! Eso*

no es nada!' ['That's nothing!'] 'How will you ever collect enough to be worth it?'... Well, no, it is not much of anything, but that is not what was most important to us. We were interested in our health and the ecology ... and that's how it was. We didn't care about the 20 cents, we just wanted to get rid of all the garbage we were seeing and improve health conditions around here. (Interviews, June 2011)

The struggles demonstrated through the stories of women who take on responsibility for community garbage management are in many ways consistent with other studies of neoliberal natural resource policies throughout Latin America that give local actors further responsibility without the power, resources, or tools necessary for management (Perrault and Martin 2005, 197). However, the women's histories also demonstrate a shift in power dynamics, and recognition of women's important role in coastal waste management. The women themselves view their work as building a better community in coastal Yucatán by promoting clean spaces, conscious behaviours, and healthy environments at the grassroots. In the women's own words:

At this point, we cannot stop collecting recyclables, because if we do, it will all end up back in the lagoons or littered on the beaches. We clean garbage off the beach, in the fishing port, and wetlands areas. We even go to many of the areas where the authorities don't. We are used to covering all the parts of town and outside it. We go to any areas where garbage is piling up ... Every year we dedicate ourselves to cleaning out and removing tons of trash from the wetlands and beaches. (Interviews, July 2012)

The labour that these women do helps community health, as well as local tourism and conservation initiatives. As women are the main constituents of community waste management in small cities of coastal Yucatán, they protect the aesthetics and environmental health in the coastal region. Residents note that with the cleaner streets, fewer people have fallen ill to dengue or other garbage-related diseases (interviews, September 2012).

Conclusions: challenging exclusionary gender norms by increasing women's participation in community sustainable development

Globally, there remains a strong tendency in environment-development policies to frame discussions of women around their vulnerabilities in relation to broader political and environmental forces (Hanson and Buechler 2015). There is also a tendency for environmental discourses to classify 'the localised other' (people and places) according to the problems they create for broader ecosystems, with the intent of directing local actors to behave in particular ways and for specific environmental goals (Ulloa 2004). Conservation interventions therefore often perpetuate socio-environmental conflicts due to over-simplification of local power relations, and categorisation of places into fixed territories that may or may not correspond to existing spatial rationalities or practices in small urban areas.

This chapter addresses the role of garbage, not only in contaminating natural or urban spaces, but also in creating social difference based on disparate expectations of who is responsible for producing and managing garbage in the small cities of the coastal wetlands. In the case of Chen Kole 'Lob and Las Costeras, women have demonstrated their collective agency and the ways in which women's knowledge and action are central to creating innovative adaptation strategies that address urban and public health issues surrounding water and waste within protected coastal environments.

Women's collective organising confronts waste-induced water, health, and development challenges in low-lying tropical coastal areas that are overlooked due to broader concerns for large-scale ecosystem protection. Women's work also promotes sustainable development and public health in growing urban areas, and helps to underscore the muddy links of urban sanitation to gendered responsibility and the exclusionary spaces of ecological restoration in the coastal wetlands.

The research contributes to feminist geography and feminist political ecology more specifically through inclusion of personal, place-based narratives that show how women's groups produced a space for urban issues and the shifting of gender roles in coastal regions dominated by conservation-based sustainable development. This research provides a critique of the particular ways that women and coastal residents are excluded from top-down development processes, and in turn, the research establishes specific ways in which women's knowledge and practices shape 'globalising' processes of conservation through grassroots management of issues that are currently excluded from policy, namely the removal and recycling of waste products from wetlands and coastal cities and promotion of community health.

Notes

1. For example, see Gregory (2009), Oehlmann *et al.* (2009), and Teuten *et al.* (2009).
2. For a study on waste and environmental justice in the context of Oaxaca City, Mexico, see Moore (2008). For a study of the gendered context of waste in Dakar, see Fredericks (2008). For several cases of recycling and poverty reduction in Latin America, see Gutberlet (2008).
3. For example, see UNDP (2017).

Notes on contributor

Anne-Marie Hanson is an Assistant Professor of Environmental Studies at the University of Illinois Springfield. Email: ahans4@uis.edu

References

Acosta-Lugo, E., D. Alonzo-Parra, M. Andrade-Hernández, D. Castillo-Tzab, J. Chablé-Santo, R. Durán, Celene Espadas-Manrique, I. Fernández-Stohanzlova, J. Fraga, E. Galicia, J.A. González-Iturbe, J. Herrera-Silveira,

J. Sosa-Escalante, G.J. Villalobos-Zapata and F. Tun-Dzul (2010) *El Plan de Conservacíon de la Eco-Región Petenes-Celestún-Palmar,* Campeche, Campeche: Pronatura Peninsula de Yucatán, A.C. Universidad Autónoma de Campeche

Baños Ramírez, Othón (2003) *Modernidad, imaginario e identitades rurales: El caso de Yucatán,* Mexico City: El Colegio de México

Batllori-Sampedro, Eduardo, José Febles-Patrón and Julio Diaz-Sosa (1999) 'Landscape change in Yucatan's northwest coastal wetlands (1948–1991)', *Human Ecology Review* 6(1): 8–20

Batllori-Sampedro, Eduardo, M. Santibáñez-Mendieta, J. Novelo-López, F. Bautista-Zúñiga, M.A. Ortiz-Pérez, D. Quezada-Domínguez, R. Vallejo-Molina, J. Lizama, A. Cataño-Pérez, O. PaviaMartín and F. Cime-López (2006) *Ordernamiento Ecológico Local del Territorio en La Reserva de la Biosfera Ría Celestún: Una Perspectiva Estructuralista,* Mérida, Yucatán: Centro de Investigación y de Estudios Avanzados del IPN Unidad Mérida

Beall, Jo (2006) 'Dealing with dirt and the disorder of development: managing rubbish in urban Pakistan', *Oxford Development Studies* 34(1): 81–97, doi:10.1080/13600810500496087

Bergmann, Melanie, Lars Gutow and Michael Klages (eds.) (2015) *Marine Anthropogenic Litter,* London: Springer

Cob Chay, José (2011) 'Acuíferos contaminados Celestún necesita $6 millones para nueva red de agua', *Diario de Yucatán,* March 16, Regiones

Cob Chay, José and Wendy Ucán Chan (2010) 'Rezago en puertos yucatecos', *Diario de Yucatán,* April 15, Regiones

Doyon, Sabrina (2008) 'La construcción social del espacio: el caso de La Reserva de la Biosfera de Rio Lagartos, Yucatán, México', in Oriol Beltran, José J. Pascual and Ismael Vaccaro (eds.) *Patrimonialización de la Naturaleza. El Marco Social de las Políticas Ambientales,* Barcelona, España: Arkulegi Antropologia Elkartea, 289–306

Fraga, Julia (2006) 'Local perspectives in conservation politics: the case of the Ría Lagartos Biosphere Reserve, Yucatán, México', *Landscape and Urban Planning* 74(3–4): 285–95

Fredericks, Rosalind (2008) 'Gender and the politics of trash in Dakar: participation, labor and the "undisciplined" woman'. Thinking Gender Papers, Los Angeles: UCLA Center for the Study of Women, University of California UC Los Angeles

García de Fuentes, Ana and Manuel Xool (2012) 'Turismo alternativo y desarrollo en la costa de Yucatán', in Gustavo Marín Guardado, Ana García de Fuentes, and Magalí Daltabuit Godás (eds.) *Turismo, globalización y sociedades locales en la península de Yucatán, México, Tenerife,* Spain: PASOS, Revista de Turismo y Patrimonio Cultural, 173–96

García de Fuentes, Ana, Manuel Xool Koh, Jorge Euán Ávila, Alfonso Munguía Gil and María Dolores Cervera Montejano (2011) 'La costa de Yucatán en la perspectiva del desarrollo turístico', *Corredor Biológico Mesoamericano México Serie Conocimientos,* Número 9 México, DF: Comisión Nacional para el Conocimiento y Uso de la Biodiversidad

Gregory, Murray R. (2009) 'Environmental implications of plastic debris in marine settings – entanglement, ingestion, smothering, hangers-on, hitch-hiking and alien invasions', *Philosophical Transactions of the Royal Society B: Biological Sciences* 364(1526): 2013–25, doi:10.1098/rstb.2008.0265

Gutberlet, Julia (2008) *Recovering Resources – Recycling Citizenship: Urban Poverty Reduction in Latin America,* Aldershot, Hants and Burlington, VT: Ashgate

Hanson, Anne-Marie (2015) 'Shoes in the seaweed and bottles on the beach: global garbage and women's oral histories of socio-environmental change in coastal Yucatán', in Stephanie Buechler and Anne-Marie Hanson (eds.) *A Political Ecology of Women, Water, and Global Environmental Change,* London: Routledge, 165–84

Hanson, Anne-Marie S. (2016) 'Women's ecological oral histories of recycling and development in coastal Yucatán', *Gender, Place & Culture* 23(4): 467–83

Hanson, Anne-Marie and Stephanie Buechler (2015) 'Towards a feminist political ecology of women, global change, and vulnerable waterscapes', in Stephanie Buechler and Anne-Marie Hanson (eds.) *A Political Ecology of Women, Water, and Global Environmental Change,* London: Routledge, 1–16

Harris, Leila (2009) 'Gender and emergent water governance: comparative overview of neoliberalized natures and gender dimensions of privatization, devolution and marketization', *Gender, Place & Culture* 16(4): 387–408, doi:10.1080/09663690903003918

INEGI (2015) *Anuario estadístico y geográfico de Yucatán,* México: Instituto Nacional de Estadística y Geografía

Jenkins, Katy (2008) 'Practically professionals? Grassroots women as local experts – a Peruvian case study', *Political Geography* 27(2): 139–59, doi:10.1016/j.polgeo.2007.07.006

Lliteras, Sentíes Eduardo (2009) 'La basura, amenaza para la salud y el turismo en Celestún', *Revista de Yucatán,* 21 July

Moore, Sarah A. (2008) 'The politics of garbage in Oaxaca, Mexico', *Society & Natural Resources* 21(7): 597–610

Moser, Caroline (1993) *Gender Planning and Development: Theory, Practice and Training,* London: Routledge

Oehlmann, J., U. Schulte-Oehlmann, W. Kloas, O. Jagnytsch, I. Lutz, K.O. Kusk, L. Wollenberger, E.M. Santos, G.C. Paull, K.J. Van Look and C.R. Tyler (2009) 'A critical analysis of the biological impacts of plasticizers on wildlife', *Philosophical Transactions of the Royal Society B: Biological Sciences* 364(1526): 2047–62, doi:10.1098/rstb.2008.0242

Perrault, Thomas and Patricia Martin (2005) 'Special issue on geographies of neoliberalism in Latin America', *Environment and Planning A* 37(2): 191–201

Rimarachín Cabrera, Isidro, Emma Zapata Martelo and Verónica Vásquez García (2001) 'Gender, rural households, and biodiversity in native Mexico', *Agriculture and Human Values* 18(1): 85–93

Robles de Benito, Rafael (2005) *Apropiación de recursos naturales y relaciones sociales en la Reserva de la Biosfera Ría Celestún, Yucatán.* Maestro en Ciencias, Ecología Humana, Centro de Investigación y de Estudios Avanzados del Instituto Politécnico Nacional, Unidad Mérida

Schwanse, Elvira (2011) 'Recycling policies and programmes for PET drink bottles in Mexico', *Waste Management & Research* 29(9): 973–81, doi:10.1177/0734242X11413331

SEDUMA (2009) *Programa Especial para la Prevención y Gestión Integral de los Residuos 2009–2012, Merida,* Yucatán: Secretaría de Desarollo Urbano y Medio Ambiente

Teuten, E. L., J. M. Saquing, D. R. Knappe, M. A. Barlaz, S. Jonsson, A. Bjorn, S. J. Rowland, R. C. Thompson, T. S. Galloway, R. Yamashita, D. Ochi, Y.

Watanuki, C. Moore, P. H. Viet, T. S. Tana, M. Prudente, R. Boonyatumanond, M. P. Zakaria, K. Akkhavong, Y. Ogata, H. Hirai, S. Iwasa, K. Mizukawa, Y. Hagino, A. Imamura, M. Saha and H. Takada (2009) 'Transport and release of chemicals from plastics to the environment and to wildlife', *Philosophical Transactions of the Royal Society B: Biological Sciences* 364(1526): 2027–45, doi:10.1098/rstb.2008.0284

Ulloa, Astrid (2004) *La construcción del nativo ecológico*, Bogotá: Instituto Colombiano de Antropología e Historia -ICANHCOLCIENCIAS

UN-OCEANS (2013) 'Human settlements on the coast', in *UN Atlas of the Oceans*, http://www.oceansatlas.org/subtopic/en/c/114/ (last checked 18 May 2017)

UNDP (2017) F*ortalecimiento de la Participación Ciudadana y Gobernanza Ambiental para la Sustentabilidad* (Strengthening Citizen Participation and Environmental Geovernance for Sustainability), http://www.mx.undp.org/content/mexico/es/home/operations/projects/environment_and_energy/fortalecimiento-de-la-participacion-ciudadana-y-gobernanza-ambie.html (last checked 18 May 2017)

UNEP (2006) *Marine Litter in the Wider Caribbean*, Kingston, Jamaica: United Nations Environment Programme – Caribbean Environment Programme

UNEP (2016) *Marine plastic debris and microplastics – Global lessons and research to inspire action and guide policy change*, Nairobi: United Nations Environment Programme

Vásquez Avila, Leidy Aurora, Saishi Ota and Carlos Mauricio Alarcón Lazcano (2011) *Manual para el Establecimiento de un Sistema de manejo de Residuos Sólidos en Ciudades, Pequeñas Comunidades Rurales y Areas Naturales Protegidas. Estudio de Caso: Municipio de Celestún, Yucatán, México, Proyecto de Conservación de Humedales en la Península de Yucatán*, Mérida, Mexico: CONANP-JICA

CHAPTER 6

Reframing women's empowerment in water security programmes in Western Nepal

*Stephanie Leder, Floriane Clement
and Emma Karki*

Abstract

Water security has become the new buzzword for water and development programmes in the rural South. The concept has potential to focus policymakers and practitioners on the inequalities and injustices that lie behind lack of access to affordable, safe, and clean water. The concept of women's empowerment also provides an opportunity to do this. However, the vast majority of water security interventions using the term are apolitically and technically framed and fail to understand complex intersectional inequalities. We suspect that many of these interventions have been implemented following a business-as-usual approach with the risk of reproducing and even exacerbating existing gendered inequalities in access to and control over water. This chapter explores these concerns in the context of four villages in Western Nepal, where two internationally funded programmes aimed to empower women by improving access to water for both domestic and productive uses. They hoped to transform women into rural entrepreneurs and grassroots leaders. However, differences between women – such as age, marital status, caste, remittance flow, and land ownership – led to some women benefiting more than others. Water programmes must recognise and address difference between women if the poorest and most disadvantaged women are to benefit. Gender mainstreaming in the water sector needs to update its understanding of women's empowerment in line with current feminist understandings of it as a processual, relational, and multi-dimensional concept. This means focusing on inter-household relations within communities, as well as intra-household relations. In addition, we recommend that water security programmes rely on more nuanced and context-specific understandings of women's empowerment that go beyond enhanced access to resources and opportunities to develop agency to include social networks, critical consciousness, and values.

Keywords: Women's empowerment; water security; multiple-use water systems; feminisation of agriculture; intersectionality; complex inequalities

http://dx.doi.org/10.3362/9781788530866.006

Introduction

International discussions, policymaking, and practice on water and development are increasingly framed around the concept of water security, defined by UN-Water (2013, iv) as

> the capacity of a population to safeguard sustainable access to adequate quantities of acceptable quality water for sustaining livelihoods, human well-being, and socio-economic development.

Mainstream international water security discourses have been criticised for their failure to consider adequately issues related to inequalities by gender, and more broadly power issues (Allouche 2011; Clement 2013).

This is interesting in light of the fact that we have seen decades of activism and progress on gender mainstreaming in development, an idea that originated over two decades ago (United Nations 1995). Gender mainstreaming sees the empowerment of women as a goal in itself, as well as an essential step in ensuring development interventions are effective and deliver their goals.

There has been enormous progress to 'mainstream' gender issues into development, and into the water sector, using various concepts and analytical tools to ensure women's gender-specific interests and needs are addressed (Cronin *et al.* 2015). Water security programmes, whether in the water, sanitation, and hygiene (WASH) or irrigation sectors, have stressed the need for women's participation in water management, and even claimed that enhanced access to water contributes to women's empowerment. Yet it is unclear how these claims can be fulfilled in the context of neoliberal approaches to water security promoting individualisation of water rights, privatisation, and marketisation (Ahlers and Zwarteveen 2009).

Women's empowerment is a holistic concept that has social and political, as well as economic, dimensions. It requires change to gendered structures of power, but also to structures of power relating to other aspects of identity including class, race, and caste. However, development programming has tended to focus on economic empowerment of individual women as an anti-poverty measure, enabling them to contribute to national economic growth but failing to challenging the current technical and managerial model of development. Development interventions and policies that focus on women's economic empowerment have been accused of using the term empowerment as a buzzword, failing to bring real economic or social change or challenge conservative gender norms (Batliwala 2007).

A broader view of women's economic empowerment in a water security perspective sees it as an essential aspect of a more holistic process of change. Naila Kabeer's conceptualisation of empowerment is a feminist view of the importance of material resources in the lives of poor women. However, in addition to support extending their access to and control over resources, women need support extending their agency. Agency could be described as the ability to make strategic decisions to achieve what one values. Women's empowerment is a complex concept, which is not only about economic change, but also about political and social change; about gender inequality, but also about other aspects of identity that women share with men, like class or caste. These other aspects of difference intersect with gender, making it difficult for particular women to take advantage of development programming aiming at enhancing water security.

Programming on water for women's empowerment: our research

In the following sections, we examine how two sister water security projects aiming to support women's empowerment in Nepal translated into practice.

The projects we focused on in our research provided interesting examples of how the issues we have raised played out in practice. The two projects clearly envisioned a linear impact pathway linking enhanced access to water to economic empowerment, which in turn was to support women's agency and leadership, and ultimately to lead to social change.

Our discussion uses Naila Kabeer's (1999) feminist view of women's empowerment to explore the links between resources and agency, and between agency and achievements. We examine the following questions: How is access to water resources linked to women's agency, and how do resources and agency translate or not into achievements and desired social change? We suspect that the linkages are non-linear contrarily to the impact pathways envisioned by the project.

In our discussion, we aim to demonstrate how women of different caste, class, and age, living in various household situations, were able to benefit differently from improved water access as a result of the two programmes we focused on. We also explored the projects' abilities to acknowledge and address how the dynamic interplay of cultural norms, gender roles, and power relations shape access to and control over water resources, particularly in the context of male emigration.

Our research was conducted as part of two development programmes implemented in the farand mid-western regions of Nepal by the same international non-government organisation, International Development Enterprises (iDE).[1] The two projects were funded by different sources.[2] We, human geographers at the International Water Management Institute in Nepal, conducted the research as project partners to analyse how the project interventions contributed to women's empowerment. As research outputs we developed a research report, and implemented and filmed a participatory gender training.[3]

Research methods

We collected data in four case study villages: Milanpur located in Kailali district (Nigali VDC), Punebata and Tiltali in Doti district (Khatiwada and Latamandu VDCs) and Silinge in Dadeldhura district (Samejee VDC) districts in Nepal's Far-Western region (Figure 1). For this study in four communities,

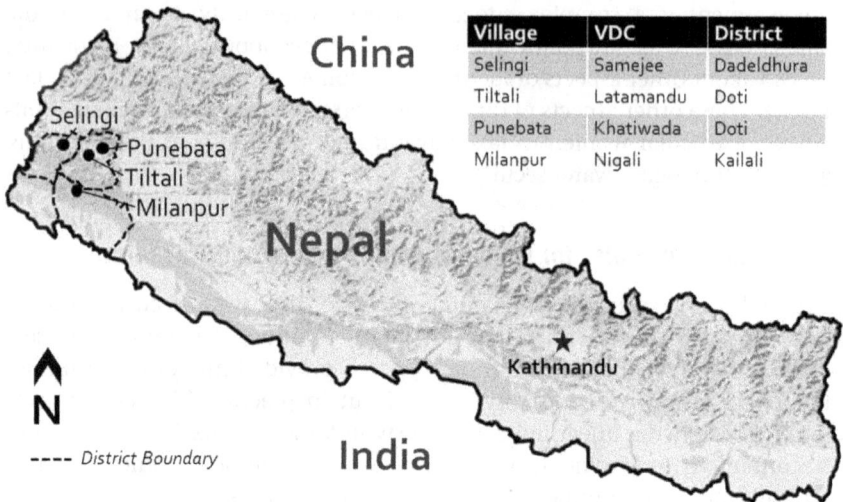

Village	VDC	District
Selingi	Samejee	Dadeldhura
Tiltali	Latamandu	Doti
Punebata	Khatiwada	Doti
Milanpur	Nigali	Kailali

Figure 1. Location of the four case study sites.

we triangulated qualitative methods such as in-depth interviews, life histories, observations and transect walks, focus group discussions with empowerment rankings, Venn diagrams, and village resource mappings, and the results of a household survey which was conducted for the purpose of the two projects' impact evaluation.

Around 70 women and 30 men were involved in our research. We held 22 focus group discussions, 44 in-depth interviews, and 16 life histories. To gain in-depth perspectives on farmers' social networks and their perceptions of the development programmes, we involved the same participants in different participatory methodologies over a period of two field visits throughout the initiation and implementation of project interventions. In addition, we were engaged as project partners in diverse inception, planning, and reporting workshops, and held formal interviews and informal discussions with project staff in the field.

Households in the case study villages consist of 17 per cent Dalits (marginalised castes, formerly referred to as 'Untouchables') and 7 per cent Janajati (indigenous nationalities), while 78 per cent of households are Brahmin, Chettri, and others considered as upper castes (Central Bureau of Statistics 2014a, 2014b, 2014c). According to the project baseline survey, 35 per cent of households in the case study villages are female-headed.

The region is marked by a high rate of long-term male out-migration to India, Malaysia, and the Gulf region, with a high dependence on remittances to manage household expenses. Households also depend on women's labour and earnings. In addition to care within the household, married women in landless households work as agricultural labourers, and if land is owned, contribute to family's farming. As the projects targeted villages accessible by road, with market access and potential for vegetable cultivation, in the villages where the programmes ran, many women already cultivated vegetables in their homestead garden prior to the project interventions. In two of the case study villages, a few women also sold their products on the market. However, very few women did vegetable farming and selling at a commercial scale – rather most of them grow for subsistence and sell the surplus, if any. The land used for kitchen gardens are small individual plots owned by their husbands and fathers-in-law.

Project aims and activities

The two projects explicitly aimed at empowering women by improving access to water for both domestic and productive uses through the construction of multiple-use water systems (MUS) (Van Koppen and Kuriakose 2009). They also supported women's involvement in small-scale commercial horticulture through horticulture training and the establishment of farmer-managed vegetable collection centres.

In the Western hills of Nepal, women's access to water resources is largely shaped by class and caste. Caste in particular often determines the location of the household within the diverse elevations of the village's area. Some communal taps existed before the project. In two of our case study villages, while upper-caste households are located in areas with higher water pressure on taps, Dalits and other traditionally marginalised households experienced more leakages and less water pressure in their communal taps, which they shared with a higher number of households than upper-caste households. On average, four to ten households shared communal taps in areas of the villages where Dalits and traditionally marginalised people lived, compared to one to four households sharing each communal tap in areas with upper-caste inhabitants.

In these villages, when water supply through the communal taps proved insufficient, women have to fetch water from *naulas* (natural water springs). However, Dalits are not allowed to touch *naulas*, due to restrictive cultural norms because it is believed that they contaminate water sources if they touch them. Consequently, in the dry season, Dalits have to wait at the *naula* for an upper-caste woman to come and fill their vessels for them. Alternatively, Dalit women fetch murky water from the river. This adds additional time, work, and ultimately emotional stress burden on Dalit women.

The MUS that the projects installed are either single-use drinking water systems, upgraded to provide additional water for small-scale commercial horticulture in homestead land, or new systems specifically designed to provide water for both domestic and productive needs. MUS are meant to reduce the time women spend fetching water for domestic uses through improved water access with a piped distribution system leading to taps, and at the same time to support women's productive engagement in vegetable farming (*ibid.*).

The MUS were installed or upgraded in each of the four villages. The aim was that every household receives a tap, although this varied across different areas of relative wealth or poverty; in some Dalit areas, housing was denser leading to as many as 15 households depending on one MUS.

In each village, social mobilisers (project staff responsible for about ten villages) formed water user groups of about 15–20 households and farmer groups with 20–25 farmers who were to receive water infrastructure and vegetable farming training. These groups consisted of interested women and men who usually had been engaged in earlier development projects which required group formations. A gender balance and the inclusion of Dalits and Janjatis, though not in concrete numbers, were given as recommendation to social mobilisers. Every group included an executive committee consisting of a president, a secretary, and a treasurer, which were decided by majority vote – that is as per the decision of the group, usually decided by one or two and supported by the rest of the group.

Several training programmes were held for each farmer group (for about 20–25 individuals per village) as part of the project to provide knowledge and skills on horticulture, nutrition, account keeping, maternal health, group management, and gender in both villages. Local partners also conducted training programmes in a demonstration garden with an irrigation drip kit in each village. A key project initiative is to establish vegetable collection centres and a marketing and planning committee to manage the centre. The centre is accessible to all farmers, irrespective of the quantity of vegetables they bring. However, due to insufficient production at the time of our fieldwork, these were not yet operational in the area of our case study villages.

Power relations, water resource access, and women's agency

In this section, we explore what our research reveals about the links between power relations, access to water, and women's agency, and consider the extent to which the projects were able to support women's empowerment. For our analysis, we build on Naila Kabeer's conceptualisation of empowerment, as

> the process by which those who have been denied the ability to make strategic life choices acquire such an ability. (Kabeer 1999, 436)

The empowerment process envisioned by both projects was based on enhancing women's agency by transforming them to become successful rural entrepreneurs through enhanced water access and capacity building, contributing to their economic empowerment and to enhanced decision-making over agricultural production, through commercial horticulture.

Naila Kabeer (1999) views empowerment as a *process* of change by expanding people's ability to make strategic decisions that result in *desired* outcomes. The ability to make strategic choices incorporates three interrelated dimensions: *agency, resources,* and *achievements.* A pre-condition to exercise choice is the access to and control over material, and human and social *resources.* As a further dimension, the *achievements* of choice must be understood in terms of well-being outcomes (e.g. nourishment, health, shelter) as this sheds light on the equality of, and not differences in, choices. The ability to define one's goals and act upon them determines someone's *agency*. However, this choice is only possible if alternative options exist, which enables the

> emergence of a critical consciousness, the process by which people move from a position of unquestioning acceptance of the social order to a critical perspective on it. (Kabeer 1999, 440)

Feminist understandings of empowerment (Rowlands 1998) focus on the importance of building a sense of personal empowerment ('power within'), which gives meaning to agency ('power to'). This sense of the importance of power within echoes the concept of *critical consciousness* (Freire 1970).

We drew on these ideas in our research, seeing it as very important in processes of empowerment to be aware of alternative ways of living, and to the consciousness of oppressive social and politic-economic structures in empowerment processes. Of particular interest to us in this study was the process of how critical consciousness and resources translate into the realisation of choices, as well as its outcomes on achievements/wellbeing. This process can also be seen as circular, as well-being outcomes can in turn influence resources as well as agency.

Intra-household power relationships

Predictably, intra-household power relationships affected women's agency, including their freedom to participate in groups and training sessions offered in the projects. However, focusing only on gender as a single category can reproduce power relations. In our case study area, agency, or the ability to make strategic decisions to achieve what one values, depends on familial support, the household composition, and one's position within the household.

Factors that were important included marital status, and the presence or not of husbands in the household (some were migrant workers and absent, as previously discussed). Other important issues included women's age, the age and number of any children, and other people including parents-in-law and other older people, and adult siblings, for example.

Gender relations in the household were clearly important. In a traditional extended family household with three generations present, women needed to seek permission from their husband or in-laws to leave household care work and attend meetings. However, gender relations were not the only important social relations which shaped women's ability to participate. Attending meetings relied not only on husbands' permission but also on the willingness and ability of another female family member to manage some domestic tasks on her behalf. Young women, in particular, were primarily responsible for household work and child care, and their ability to expand their agency critically depended on the labour and emotional support from other female family members, including the mother-in-law.

A daughter-in-law mentioned that she had to seek not only her husband's permission to attend training sessions, but also her mother-in-law's support to manage the household in her absence. She said:

> If the mother-in-law helps out with the household work then we can go and attend training. If the husband allows us to go, then we can go. (Focus group discussion, Tiltali, Latamandu VDC, Doti district, November 2015)

A particularly important point to note in the context of projects aiming to promote the empowerment of women in the region is that particularly in the absence of men due to migration, mothers-in-law often largely shaped the agency of their daughters-in-law, and notably their involvement in water and development projects.

These insights show the power hierarchies due to age and family position in female relations, and confirm that women's empowerment – both as an outcome and a process – is affected by their relationships with other women as well as with men. We have to take an intersectional perspective and look not only at the category 'gender', but at power relations, if we are to understand the empowering potential of a development project in a particular context.

Women who had taken up leadership positions in the water-user groups and vegetable farming groups formed by the projects noted that encourage-ment by their husbands or mothers-in-law was essential in their decisions to go ahead, as emphasised by a female farmer in Kailali:

> When we held meetings, all husbands said: 'my wife cannot do it' [being in the executive committee]. I received a lot of help from my husband. My husband proposed me and first I said no but he said 'you will be fine'. (Interview, Milanpur community, Nigali VDC, Kailali, October 2015)

Changes in household form were also important. Male out-migration in this context had clearly greatly affected intra-household relationships and intra-household bargaining on water resource access. Alongside increasing male emigration, another social change affecting families and households is occurring within these communities. Many households are moving to a nuclear family set-up, meaning that the young couples live apart from the husband's parents. When husbands are absent working, young women are heading the household. The issue of seeking permission from in-laws is thus resolved to an extent once the extended family set-up is dismantled. As a result, some young women are able to set their own work schedule and make decisions independently, including regarding their participation in water user group meetings, whereas others still have to seek for their husband's permis-sion through phone calls.

Overall, we found that the increase in nuclear households and male out-migration are both contributing to challenge the traditionally defined role of wife and mother in which husbands and parents-in-law all expect young women to remain within the household. Increasingly, young women were stepping into the public sphere. As a direct effect of male emigration, women have gained visibility and received opportunity to occupy spaces previously reserved for men. For instance, in the case of water user groups, which require one member per household, women from female-headed households are representing their households. But in extended families, this opportunity would not arise in the same way: a father-in-law or mother-in-law might attend meetings, and young women would have less opportunity to challenge traditional gender norms.

Beyond gender relations to intersectionality: caste and class affect women's empowerment

Within the hills of Far-Western Nepal, where settlements are spread over a rugged terrain, the MUS often only benefits a small group within a larger community, which leads to equity concerns. Across our four case study villages, we observed that mostly households of the affluent and politically connected benefited from the project water intervention. As discussed earlier, before the projects, villages were dependent either on communal taps or on water from springs, and access to taps was much better for households with class and caste advantages. Whereas the two projects' interventions also benefited Dalit villages, we found that in the case of mixed-caste communities, the projects largely did not tackle the fact that households did not have the same ability to access water within their community.

In both traditional and externally supported water systems, the distribution of water across households in a given community has often been determined by the local elite and powerful. A planned development project should therefore seek transparent mechanisms to ensure universal access and address problems of unequal provision. Upon project field staff entering villages to select and form groups of beneficiaries, local power and geographical asymmetries came into play to shape project outcomes. Those within the community who were most outspoken and politically connected, mostly male Chettri or Brahmin leaders, were the entry points for the project into the community. They provided the project with information on the community's water needs and helped project staff to organise village meetings by informing other villagers.

In Milanpur, for instance, the MUS was located in the vicinity of the political leader's house, serving his house and nine other houses in a village of 50 households. Similarly, in Punebata and Punetola, some of the taps and thai jars were located near the homes of the already more successful vegetable farmers who are growing vegetables at a relatively larger scale compared to the rest of the village and who bought drip kits from the project. In the case study site Silinge, the secretary of the water user group formed by the project, an outspoken woman from an upper caste, who had the knowledge and network to reach out to project staff, received a second tap in her garden just by requesting the project officer:

> I checked the list and my name was not there so I called the office and told them I need a tap. If my garden is used as a demo garden then I also need a [second] tap. (Interview, Silinge, Samajee VDC, Dadeldhura district, May 2016)

Despite the projects' intentions to include Dalits and women in meetings and in decisionmaking processes related to project implementation, the lack of consideration of the subtleties and complexities of intersectional power relations led to counter-productive results. For instance, as staff were informed to include Dalits and women, they often selected female Dalits. This resulted in meetings with Chettri men and Dalit women, which created a 'double barrier' for Dalit women to express their views and influence the decision-making process. Hence, their agency, the ability to make and influence decisions on which taps and sources would be upgraded or on the location of installing new taps, was restricted, as their participation was tokenistic, and they were unable to influence decision-making.

In the village of Silinge, Dalit villagers reported that the decision on the location of individual taps was already made prior to the community meeting and that Dalit requests were simply overlooked. As a result, in the village with 59 Chettri and nine Dalit households, only one out of 23 taps installed by the project were given to a Dalit household. The selected Dalit household resides apart from the other Dalits near the community leader's house at the top of the village. The Dalits who openly requested a tap were told that they already have one, although they share it with more households than upper castes, and although it is regularly blocked and malfunctioning. Despite the project's intention, the Dalits were further marginalised and put in a more vulnerable position. They still have to frequent the *naula* but fewer Chettri women are around to help them fill their vessels, because they now have access to private taps.

To sum up, those with influence and well-connected were able to negotiate in their favour using their position of power. Furthermore, these farmers were able to additionally benefit from access to water by also receiving a range of related project interventions such as horticulture and nutrition training, drip irrigation kits, mulching drums, and seed provisions. They were able to further build on these material, social, and human resources to use their improved access to water to engage in commercial horticulture enterprises.

This is not to say that the projects only benefited upper-caste and powerful households. In another case study site, the MUS benefited a Dalit female-headed household but did not reach some powerful Chettri households. Our point is that who benefited and who did not was left to local power relationships and existing social and geographical inequalities in accessing water, in the absence of a transparent planning process and a strategy to include the most disempowered and marginalised groups of the village.

Agency does not equal achievements

Meanings and values

We examined earlier how power relationships affect women's access to water resources, their ability to benefit from access to resources, and their agency. In Naila Kabeer's framework, agency is linked to values. We now look at the links between increased individual agency of women, and their achievements, giving particular attention to the meanings and values women attached to material and social resources such as water, land, and seeds, as well as family relations. In particular, we critically reflect on the extent to which individual forms of agency envisioned by international water security discourses resonate with women's values in our case study area.

In two of our case study sites, in Nigali and Khatiwada VDCs, many young women were able to engage in small-scale commercial horticulture, thanks to increased and more reliable access to water close to their home. Many women informants reported they enjoyed vegetable gardening and were satisfied to have some cash at their disposal from the vegetables sales, which they used to buy basic household items or pay school fees. It relieved them from the stress of asking their mother-in-law or husband for some petty cash.

According to our observations in the case study villages, however, this did not translate into a transformative change in status for women. Apart from a few exceptional cases, vegetable sales still provided a secondary source of income for the household, which was not sufficient for young daughters-in-law to increase their bargaining power – their husbands were still the main breadwinner. This extra economic income could come with high physical burden and time-intensive walks to markets for women, a task that no men would have accepted to do, as they found it was a woman's job which was degrading for men (Clement and Karki in press).

Furthermore, local women did not necessarily perceive individual agency as contributing to well-being. For example, we encountered one landless Dalit woman in the village of Tiltali. She is an outspoken community member who shares her opinion confidently, and makes decisions independently in the absence of her migrated husband. Yet she reported continuous emotional stress. She expressed the view that it is not desirable to make all the decisions in the household, and that she would have preferred to discuss and decide with her husband.

Her narrative demonstrates a recurring case we encountered during our field work: it is neither valued nor socially desirable for women to make decisions individually, rather it is culturally valued to seek acceptance and support by in-laws and husbands. This is in opposition to projects' assumption that solely individual decision-making at the household level means empowerment. Hence, individuals have to be viewed as embedded within the household as a co-operative unit because individual's empowerment is highly dependent on relations with husbands and in-laws. Therefore, approaches have to engage other household members, e.g. by encouraging the participation of daughters-in-law in training.

This finding confirms that empowerment is differently connotated by the women whom the development seeks to support than by outsiders – a point made by Naila Kabeer in the context of an analysis of women in Bangladesh and their experience of microfinance projects in the 1990s (Kabeer 2001).

Local perceptions of empowerment

To disentangle the local perceptions that meaningful and contextualised water security programmes need to take into account, we explored farmers' perceptions and values of empowerment using in-depth interviews and life histories. In a participatory process, women brought up a range of issues discussing *shashaktikaran* (empowerment in Nepali).

At first, both Chettri and Dalit women stressed the centrality of access to resources and, in particular, land and water, to become empowered farmers. However, as the discussion progressed, they brought up issues related to Kabeer's dimension of agency. They highlighted the need of a supportive husband and family for a woman to be able to become an empowered farmer, together with personal characteristics such as hard work, courage, skills, and knowledge.

> Empowered women have a good and supportive family, they are respected and know their rights. (Focus group discussion, Silinge, Samajee VDC, Dadeldhura district, May 2016)

A striking example was a woman from an upper caste, who runs the household and the farm alone as her husband is disabled. She and her family live separately from the inlaws, which is still rather unusual in her community. She is outspoken and engaged in community activities. Her garden was selected by the project to set up as demonstration plot for horticulture and MUS, and she also became the leader of one of the farmer groups created by the project. Despite a challenging household situation, she demonstrated a critical consciousness of her own situation and could assemble women in the village to discuss the progress of water interventions.

She closely communicated with the social mobiliser working on the project, who provided her firsthand information to pass on to other women and negotiate with them the location of water taps. This case demonstrates the reciprocal relationship of agency and resources: agency leads to better water resource access, which in turn contributes to improved agency.

This example and the quotation demonstrate the fuzzy interconnectedness of water resources, agency, and achievements in Naila Kabeer's framework. Women attribute high value to familial and communal support and knowledge sharing in order to improve their water access. This highlights that intangible aspects, such as supportive social relations and self-confidence, are explicitly linked to the ability to benefit from improved water access. It points to the need for water security programmes to create spaces in which diverse male and female farmers can share and discuss with project staff what they value, which can in turn be integrated into the design and implementation of technical training and water interventions.

Conclusion and recommendations from our research

We have explored feminist understandings of women's empowerment, and focused in particular on the contrast between them and the narrower under-standings of economic empowerment that currently inform many develop-ment projects. In our study of water security interventions, we used insights from Naila Kabeer's framework of empowerment to analyse the extent to which these interventions offered scope to women to increase access to water resources and build agency, to achieve significant change that is valuable to them. Our analysis highlighted that the relationships linking water resource development and women's empowerment are complex and highly location- and household specific.

On the one hand, we showed that individual women's empowerment is shaped by power relationships at the community level and beyond, particu-larly in relation to project staff from outside. On the other hand, empower-ment has to be understood within the broader household relations marked by ages, household composition, one's position in the household, and intra-familial support. Our study demonstrates that these interand intra-household relations of different kinds – including caste, age, and family positioning – have to be taken into account when aiming at empowering 'women' through water security interventions, as these shape who and how one can gain and benefit from enhanced access to water resources and expand one's agency.

Local meanings and values attributed to empowerment are important to understand and flexibly address in the design of water security programmes to work more effectively towards social change. In our case study areas, the meanings and values that diverse women attributed to empowerment indicate that individual decision-making is culturally not desired, and that household support is necessary before participating in training and group meetings of water security projects. Hence, interventions should take social relationships into account and not necessarily oppose women's agency to men's agency. This is even more important in the context of changing gender relations in households and communities due to male emigration.

Such a relational framing of empowerment has important implications for water security project design, implementation, monitoring, and evaluation: it needs to take intersectionality and the social networks within which diverse women act into account. Considering intersectionality is also important to avoid applying one single model of empowerment pathway on all villages and women. We reckon that our approach to empowerment touches upon broader issues about the ways water and development projects are framed. The latter are largely driven by results-based agendas and logical frame approaches which tend to reproduce simplistic and apolitical conceptualisations of empowerment. Adopting a rela-tional framing of empowerment therefore also means that the different actors acknowledge the political and social dimensions of the issues they want to address not only in their projects, but also within their own organisations.

Hence, in contrast to the dominant narrow and instrumentalist framing of empowerment adopted in water security programmes, we argue for a more relational and processual framing of empowerment that engages with structural and social change.

To conclude, we offer a few recommendations for moving in this direction. Given the changing social conditions, water security programmes can strengthen women's increasing agency when being sensitive to their time schedules and also involving other family members to convince them to support their wives and daughters-in-law. Hence, the success of the programme in empowering women lies in the ability to consider intra-household relationships and the differentiated abilities women have to expand their agency depending on their household situation.

In addition, water security interventions need to consider shifting divisions of labour and agricultural practices, as well as changing gendered norms in water resource management. We suggest a rigorous gender analysis in each project at the planning stage to develop implementation and uptake approaches which allow the maximum potential for increasing women's agency over water resources by identifying: how can the project develop a better understanding of intra-household and intra-community power relations and design water interventions based on contextualised meanings of empowerment?

This would require a broader framing beyond economic empowerment, with both quantitative and qualitative survey methods. It would also mean that different beneficiary categories are designed according to the local context. For example, in the case of Nepal, we see three to four important intersecting categories disaggregated by gender, age, caste/ethnicity, and/or class. Accordingly, projects could design specific interventions to approach individuals from these categories, for instance, young men (sensitising for gender issues, involving in programmes as they otherwise become future migrants), young daughters-in-law (child care as incentives), female-headed households (adjusting timings and reducing work burden), or landless/Dalit women (provide interventions that do not require land ownership). For this, we defend the need to go beyond technical feasibility surveys, to also integrate assessment of social inequalities and, in particular, how multiple social markers intersect to shape access to water within local communities.

Therefore, we argue for creating more space and a supportive environment for flexible grassroots implementation processes. Water security programmes, before intervening technically, could integrate capacity development and confidence-building approaches for collective empowerment, focusing on capturing and addressing diverse men and women's critical consciousness and values on empowerment. In addition to technical training and infrastructural provisions, diverse community members should have space to discuss meaningful approaches to include the most marginalised households. Such a participatory and contextualised design of project interventions gives space for developing bottom-up approaches, which are initially more time and human resource intense, but may be more sustainable afterwards. Examples are participatory training aiming at raising critical consciousness on gender inequality by explicitly encouraging communities to discuss genderand caste-based discrimination in their villages, and by motivating them to find solutions collectively for more inclusive project implementation processes which target a range of beneficiaries of diverse backgrounds (Leder *et al.* 2016).

Finally, participatory gender training for field staff and farmers can be an effective way to sensitise them on individuals' and households' differential water resource access and agency. To provide space for developing a critical consciousness and self-confidence, we suggest discussing values with farmer groups. This can help by taking local cultural norms into account to develop meaningful and contextualised approaches to women's empowerment.

Notes

1. For further information on iDE and its programmes, see www.ideglobal.org and, for its work in Nepal, see www.idenepal.org (last checked 6 June 2017).
2. One programme was funded by the United States Agency for International Development (USAID) and the other programme was funded by UK's Department for International Development (DFID) programme BRACED (Building Resilience and Adaptation to Climate Extremes and Disasters).
3. The unpublished research report for the BRACED-Anukulan project is by the authors of this chapter and is entitled 'Linking Women's Empowerment and Their Resilience'. The participatory gender training conducted has been published by Leder *et al.* (2016). A film documentary, webinar slides, and an interactive homepage of the implemented training can be found at https://wle.cgiar.org/solutions/participatory-gender-training-community-groups (last checked 6 June 2017).

Acknowledgements

We would like to thank the Department for International Development programme BRACED (Building Resilience and Adaptation to Climate Extremes and Disasters) for funding our research as part of the Anukulan project 'Developing Climate Resilient Livelihoods for Local Communities Through Public– Private Partnership for 500,000 Poor People in Western Nepal that Suffer from Climate Extremes and Disasters', as well as the United States Agency for International Development for funding our research in the project 'Market Access and Water Technology for Women'. Further, we would like to thank iDE Nepal for creating a space for our research within their projects and for their logistical and technical support during our fieldwork.

Notes on contributors

Stephanie Leder is a Post-Doctoral Fellow for Gender, Youth and Social Inclusion for the CGIAR Research Program 'Water, Land and Ecosystems' (WLE) at the International Water Management Institute (IWMI) in Kathmandu, Nepal. Email: steffi.leder@gmail.com

Floriane Clement is Senior Researcher and Gender Focal Point at the International Water Management Institute (IWMI) in Kathmandu, Nepal. Email: f.clement@cgiar.org

Emma Karki is Senior Research Officer at the International Maize and Wheat Improvement Center (CIMMYT) in Kathmandu, Nepal. Email: e.karki@cgiar.org

References

Ahlers, Rhodante and Margreet Z. Zwarteveen (2009) 'The water question in feminism: water control and gender inequities in a neo-liberal era', *Gender, Place & Culture* 16(4): 409–26

Allouche, Jeremy (2011) 'The sustainability and resilience of global water and food systems: political analysis of the interplay between security, resource scarcity, political systems and global trade', *Food Policy* 36(Supplement 1): S3–S8

Batliwala, Srilatha (2007) 'Taking the power out of empowerment – An experiential account', *Development in Practice* 17(4-5): 557–65

Central Bureau of Statistics (2014a) *National Population and Housing Census 2011 (Village Development Committee/Municipality), Dadeldhura*, Kathmandu: Government of Nepal, Central Bureau of Statistics

Central Bureau of Statistics (2014b) *National Population and Housing Census 2011 (Village Development Committee/Municipality)*, Doti, Kathmandu: Government of Nepal, Central Bureau of Statistics

Central Bureau of Statistics (2014c) *National Population and Housing Census 2011 (Village Development Committee/Municipality), Kailali*, Kathmandu: Government of Nepal, Central Bureau of Statistics

Clement, Floriane (2013) 'From water productivity to water security: a paradigm shift?' in Bruce A. Lankford, Karen Bakker, Mark Zeitoun and Declan Conway (eds.) *Water Security: Principles, Perspectives and Practices*, London: Earthscan Publications, 148–65

Clement, Floriane and Emma Karki (in press) 'When water security programmes seek to empower women: case study from Western Nepal', in Christiane Fröhlich, Giovanna Gioli, Francesca Greco and Roger Cremades (eds.) *Water Security Across the Gender Divide*, Basel: Springer International Publishing

Cronin, Aidan A., Pradeep K. Mehta and Anjal Prakash (2015) *Gender Issues in Water and Sanitation Programmes: Lessons from India*, New Delhi: SAGE Publications

Freire, Paulo (1970) *Pedagogy of the Oppressed*, New York: Herder and Herder

Kabeer, Naila (1999) 'Resources, agency, achievements: reflections on the measurement of women's empowerment', *Development and Change* 30(3): 435–64

Kabeer, Naila (2001) 'Conflicts over credit: Re-Evaluating the empowerment potential of loans to women in rural Bangladesh', *World Development* 29(1): 63–84

Leder, Stephanie, Dipika Das, Andrew Reckers and Emma Karki (2016) *Participatory Gender Training for Community Groups. A Manual for Critical Discussions on Gender Norms, Roles and Relations*, Colombo, Sri Lanka: CGIAR Research Program on Water, Land and Ecosystems (WLE)

Rowlands, Jo (1998) 'A word of the times, but what does it mean? Empowerment in the discourse and practice of development', in Haleh Afshar (ed.) *Women and Empowerment: Illustrations from the Third World*, London: Macmillan, 11–34

United Nations (UN) (1996) *Report of the Fourth World Conference on Women, Beijing 4-15 September 1995*, New York: UN, http://www.un.org/women-watch/daw/beijing/pdf/Beijing%20full%20report%20E.pdf (last checked 6 June 2017)

UN-Water (2013) *UN-Water Analytical Brief on Water Security and the Global Water Agenda*, Hamilton: UNU

Van Koppen, Barbara and Anne Kuriakose (2009) 'Gender and multiple-use water services', in *Gender in Agriculture Sourcebook*, Washington, DC: World Bank, 235–41

CHAPTER 7

In troubled waters: water commodification, law, gender, and poverty in Bangalore

Kaveri Thara

Abstract

The project of privatisation of water has been floated in Bangalore since 1999, and though it has been kept in abeyance by social activists and non-government organisations working with the urban poor, water is being commoditised. In this chapter, I examine the impact of this process on the struggles of poor women to access water for themselves and their dependants, in a slum rehabilitation area in Bangalore. Women are resisting the monetisation of water, which they consider to be a human right. While the advantages of the technologies that accompany this process are emphasised by the authorities – piped water is seen as saving time and increasing mobility, as well as delivering a higher-quality resource – women retort that the requirement to pay for water outweighs any benefits, and other material realities of life still bind them to their homes.

Keywords: Water; commodification; law; legality; gender; poverty

Introduction

The project of privatisation of water has been floated in Bangalore since 1999, and though it has been kept in abeyance by social activists and NGOs working with the urban poor, water is being commercialised and commoditised. In this chapter, I draw on ethnographic research with women living in poverty in a slum rehabilitation area in the city, to examine the impact of the privatisation process on their lives. I examine women's experiences in the context of a discussion of the state's policies around water provision. Due to the sexual division of labour, women are primarily responsible for ensuring adequate water for their families, and water policies therefore have a significant impact on them. However, women in poverty are most marginalised from the policymaking processes and decisions that determine access to water in the slums of the city.

As I show here, the discussions around privatisation have framed the notion of free water as 'inadequate' and as a 'poor service', and projected paid water as enhancing health, hygiene, sanitation, efficiency, and the freedom

http://dx.doi.org/10.3362/9781788530866.007

and mobility of women. However, as my research reveals, these ideas and values are rejected by urban poor women who resist the monetisation of water, asserting instead that they have a right to access water freely, due to their poverty. They also reject the idea that freedom and mobility can increase as a result of the privatisation of water provision, pointing to the other material realities that bind them to their homes and neighbourhoods.

In the next two sections, I provide a context for my discussion, giving information on rights and water provision in India, and the history of water provision in Bangalore. I focus on recent changes in the approach taken, aiming to recover costs and involve both the private sector and individual city-dwellers in meeting the cost of water provision. I then focus on my research in Laggere, before concluding with some insights for policymakers and practitioners.

The context: rights and water provision in India

India's National Water Policies of 1987, 2002, and 2012 all recognise the human need for water, prioritising drinking water before all other water uses. However, all these policies lack a language of rights, and frame water as a basic need. Though the Indian Constitution does not specifically provide for the right to sufficient, safe, accessible, and affordable water, the right to water has been interpreted by the Supreme Court of India as well as several High Courts in India to form part of Chapter 21 which provides for the 'Right to Life'.[1] In legal cases questioning inadequate water supply in various cities in India, several legal rulings have evolved (through interpretation) the right to drinking water, which is a right that cannot be denied on the grounds of paucity of funds. It is accepted that if lack of money prevents someone from accessing safe drinking water, this would violate Chapter 21.[2]

The draft National Water Framework Bill of 2016 is meant to provide a model bill for states, and acknowledges the right of every person to:

> sufficient quantity of safe water for life within easy reach of the household regardless of, among others, caste, creed, religion, community, class, gender, age, disability, economic status, land ownership and place of residence. (Chapter 2, Chapter 3.1)

Chapter 3.3 further provides that this right shall remain, even when water service provision is delegated to a private agency.

However, financing water provision in India's ever-growing cities is an enormous challenge. In recent years, there has been a gradual reduction in India's central government budgetary allocations and guarantees for public investments, with funding deficits in the government's five-year plans, which has placed the burden of urban infrastructure investments squarely on states (Ranganathan *et al.* 2009). This presents a challenge of the idea of universal provision of water which is free to all at the point of use.

The issue of 'reforms' to the mechanisms for urban water supply and sanitation in cities of the global South have attracted interest from the World

Bank, the United States Agency for International Development (USAID), and the Asian Development Bank. The private sector is seen as a potential partner in development, including the provision of water infrastructure.[3] Public services are increasingly becoming new sites for private investment in countries across the global South.

In India, a range of strategies have aimed to help the state recover the costs of water provision. These have included encouraging more private-sector participation in water supply. Privatisation as a strategy was suggested in January 1999 by the Special Subject Group on Infrastructure formed by the Prime Minister's Council on Trade and Industry, in its report on Urban Water and Sewerage.[4] Alternative means of financing water provision are being tested via municipal bonds,[5] loans from international financial institutions, and contributions from users themselves (Ranganathan *et al.* 2009). These new forms of financing are accompanied by reforms at the municipal level such as those ushered in under the Jawaharlal Nehru National Urban Renewal Mission that aims to make cities more 'investor-friendly', in order to leverage additional funds for infrastructure and basic services (Government of India 2005).

The situation in Bangalore

In the state of Karnataka, where Bangalore lies, infrastructure for water and sanitation has historically been provided by the state government, and managed locally by municipal corporations and local governments. The city's municipal area is the Bruhat Bengaluru Mahanagara Palike, which currently spans around 800 km[2]. Public taps/fountains were the main source of water and accounted for one-third (34 per cent) of Bangalore's total water consumption in 1998 (Lele *et al.* 2013, 18).

Water provision in poor areas of the city is a complex issue.[6] Most of Bangalore's urban poor were accessing water provided by the Bangalore Water Supply and Sewerage Board (BWSSB),[7] either through public taps, or via illegal connections. Slums and squatter settlements that are notified (that is, categorised) as 'slums' are subject to the local slum laws, and have a legal right to have water provided. Most often this obligation is met by public taps installed by the local slum board. However, only a small minority of slums and squatter settlements are notified. In Bangalore, out of a total 618 slums identified by the Karnataka Slum Development Board (KDSB) (Rao 2016, n.p.), only 387 slums are notified (KDSB 2016).

In contrast, slums that are not notified have no legal right to water, and often depend on securing support from local municipal councillors and local elected members of the legislative assembly to negotiate access. In the research I focus on later, this kind of negotiation had taken place. Slums and squatter settlements are frequently demolished and the inhabitants evicted, most often from the inner-city areas, on the grounds of modernisation and development (e.g. many slums were evicted for the construction of the Bangalore Metro between 2009 and 2011 (*Express News Service* 2011, n.p.). Some of those evicted are provided rehabilitation, most often in the peripheries of the city, and most of these 'rehabilitations' do not include access to water, sanitation, and electricity.

In 2005, an informal estimate by the Karnataka Kolegeri Nivasigala Samyuktha Sanghatane (KKNSS) (a state federation of slum-dwellers) put the number of illegal slum water connections as between 20,000 and 30,000 (KKNSS 2005, cited in Wadhawan and Sharma 2007, 3). The same survey estimated 15,000 public taps were supplied by the BWSSB network, with another 3,000 supplied from local boreholes (*ibid.*).

Of the estimated 15,000 public taps provided by the BWSSB, only around 7,000 were billed to the city corporation (Connors 2005, 210). The price paid for this water was well below the actual cost of water supply, but even so, significant arrears were accumulated, standing at 15,000,000 Indian rupees (INR) by 2002 (Connors and Brocklehurst 2006, 8). The taps that went unbilled – around 8,000 – were either unauthorised or deemed to be out of service, though in practice they were still functioning (*ibid.*). Thus, an estimated 20 per cent of the water provided by the BWSSB was provided free (*ibid.*).

What was earlier viewed as a justified loss in revenue to the water authorities that would be compensated by the city corporation, in the interest of the health and hygiene of the urban poor, was now questioned. This was due to pressure on public finances in the context of rapid urbanisation, declining funding for public services, and a global development model which is still focusing on efficiency and focusing on the role of private-sector actors to substitute for a developmental state.

Watering down rights? Water privatisation in Banglalore

With the objectives of ensuring a sustainable way of resourcing water in the city, and quelling discontent from both residents and political representatives, the solution of connecting the urban poor to paid water was proposed by the Water and Sanitation Programme of the World Bank in 2000 (Connors and Brocklehurst 2006, 9).

In response to deteriorating state finances and the low capacity of municipalities to invest in infrastructure, Karnataka has been one of the most active in seeking alternative sources of financing water, and evolving efficiency savings and reforms. The project of privatisation of water was first mooted in Bangalore in 1999 (Menon 2001), and though it has been kept in abeyance for some time by social activists and NGOs working with the urban poor, the commoditisation of water has now begun.

Karnataka's Urban Drinking Water and Sanitation Policy (Government of Karnataka 2003) articulated the state's intention to carry out preparatory work to lay the ground for increased private-sector participation, including a commitment to fostering a culture of commercialisation, encouraging outsourcing, building local capacity, and most importantly identifying and expediting the necessary legislative institutional and financing changes that are necessary for private-sector participation, e.g. using tariffs. It also voices the intention of the state to recover the full cost of providing services from the users of water, together with the longer-term objective of establishing an appropriate cost-recovery mechanism through adequate tariffs, to ensure revenue for operations, maintenance costs, and servicing debt already incurred in water provision.

Significantly, the Policy also aimed to achieve 'a reasonable return on capital' (Government of Karnataka 2003, 4). As Karen Piper reveals in her compelling research on the commodification of water around the world, the language of water provision is increasingly transforming into a language of privatisation that is ushered in as enabling efficiency, pricing, and recovery of costs, thus putting a price on thirst (Piper 2015).

In 2002, the BWSSB decided to close down all public taps. The urban poor in Bangalore protested against this decision, raising many issues including the installation costs and monthly payments for water that they cannot afford. Experiences of other slum-dwellers in other parts of the city, who were issued huge monthly bills after connecting to paid water, also made them apprehensive of accepting paid connections. They requested a reduction both in installation costs and monthly payments for the urban poor, and also an assurance that the urban poor would be protected from future hikes in the price of water. The KKNSS organised a protest at the BWSSB head office on 9 May 2003. The KKNSS suggested that installation costs be fixed at no more that INR 300 and monthly tariff be at a subsidised rate of INR 50 for up to 15,000 litres a month, with protection from future price hikes.

The BWSSB has gradually phased out public taps since 2002 to reduce 'unaccounted water', while at the same time improving access to private connections (Lele *et al.* 2013). AusAID, in partnership with the BWSSB, tested paid water connections in three slums (Cement Huts, Sudamnagar, and Chandranagar) converting free water to paid connections. To make these connections possible, the BWSSB relaxed its regulations requiring documents proving legal ownership. On successfully connecting these slums, it was decided that the urban poor were 'willing to pay' for water (Wadhawan and Sharma 2007).

The Greater Bangalore Water and Sanitation Project (GBWSP), which began in 1998, is a market-based pooled finance model, adopted as a commercially viable model of water and sanitation delivery (Ranganathan *et al.* 2009). The GBWSP provides piped water to previously unconnected parts of the city, to individual homes. It recovers costs via payments from water users.

However, the policy of cost recovery has not been applied equally to all. While residents in new peripheral areas (where poverty is higher) have been expected to make payments for water, more centrally located residents in older areas of the city have not been expected to pay similarly (*ibid.*). As C.K. Prahalad and Allen Hammond revealed in research published in 2002, at that time the residents of Dharavi (a slum area in western Bangalore) paid US$1.12 per cubic metre of water – 37 times the price paid by upper-class city-dwellers who paid US$0.03 per cubic metre (Prahalad and Hammond 2002). This is because the poor have to rely on informal arrangements to obtain water, including buying water from the open market from trucks that transport water, buying drinking water from neighbouring homes for a payment per pot of water, etc. The inability of the poor to access piped water directly from the state becomes a business opportunity for others who see a profit in selling water. The provision of paid water connections is thus argued as reducing the monetary costs that the urban poor otherwise have to bear and increasing the efficiency of the BWSSB in terms of cost recovery, as well as the provision of better-quality water. The language of cost efficiency has thus replaced the language of rights.

Many slum-dwellers in Bangalore are continuing to struggle to access water free of charge, demanding water as a right, and refusing to submit to its transformation into a commodity. The shift to cost recovery is challenging assumptions about the relationship of people to water, and the obligations of the city to its inhabitants to guarantee their basic rights. Authorised access to free water is now being increasingly seen as accessing 'illegal' or 'unauthorised' connections that ushers in a new consumer relationship between the BWSSB and citizens of Bangalore. Yet the enormous significance of this change has gone largely unacknowledged.

In public communications, providing paid water connections to the poor has been characterised as 'pro poor', and depicted as providing water to slums, as if it was not provided before (Connors 2005). This ignores the fact that the urban poor have for a long time been provided free water by the BWSSB. The transformation of a right to a commodity is hailed as the ushering in of 'new working relations' between NGOs, residents, and the BWSSB, as they 'learn to cooperate and bargain with each other' (*ibid.*, 217).

In the following section, I present my research in Laggere, a slum rehabilitation area in Bangalore that consists of about 53 acres of land in the south-west of Bangalore, between 2009 and 2015, examining the struggles of urban poor women in this rapidly changing context. The research that I draw on here included interviews with 50 women residing in different neighbourhoods, 11 interviews with staff of NGOs, four focus group discussions with 24 other residents, five interviews with local leaders, apart from several conversations, and discussions with other residents in the area over a total of 13 months, spanning six years between 2009 and 2015.

Poor water: the situation in Laggere rehabilitation area

When I first visited Laggere in 2009, I was invited to participate in a group meeting organised by Priya, a resident who also co-ordinated the work of an NGO. The discussions during this meeting concerned the political accountability of the municipal councillor, as well as the role of Priya herself. She had negotiated with the elected candidate prior to his elections, trading support from the area in the form of votes in exchange for the supply of water (for a discussion on the challenges of mobilising for access to water and other services in neighbourhoods, see Haritas 2013).

During these discussions, it became clear that water was the most pressing issue for residents of Laggere, as the women and the sole man gathered in this meeting got into a heated discussion on the lack of accountability of the councillor, who had not visited the neighbourhood since his election, after having provided water connections that now did not work.

Slum housing began to be constructed in Laggere in the early 1980s by the Karnataka Slum Development Board (KSDB), to take in people who had been displaced from slum clearance elsewhere in the city. The earliest reha-bilitations to this area took place in 1983. Badly constructed apartments were handed over, lacking water, electricity, or sanitation. As the residents of these apartments do not have property titles in their names and because water connections cannot be obtained without a legal title, the KSDB as the legal owner was responsible for applying for connections. Since water connections involve payment of installation and a monthly user fee, both the KSDB and the residents organised other modes of access as nei-ther wanted to bear these costs. Rajarajeshwari Nagar ward, which houses Laggere, was previously a City Municipal Corporation area, and borewells were considered the best solution (interview with a KSDB member of staff, 26 December 2012).

However, in 2007, the ward became part of the Bangalore Municipal Corporation (Bruhat Bengaluru Mahanagara Palike) as part of Greater Bangalore, and the KSDB was now considering approaching the BWSSB, which is responsible for supplying water to Greater Bangalore and was then planning the fifth phase to connect areas added to Greater Bangalore in 2007 (Menezes 2015).

During my field work in Laggere several years after the decision, accessing water had become very difficult. Many of the public taps in the area had been removed, and some of them were locked and were to be operated for not more than one hour each day. These taps were prevented from being removed by the local councillor, who had informally negotiated limited access to water through them, during the day. In an interview with the councillor (6 January 2012), he explained that he paid a few of the area leaders a monthly stipend to operate these taps. With the reduction in taps, the amounts of water people could access had drastically fallen, with residents speaking fondly of earlier times, when they could access between 10 and 15 pots a day while now they could not access more than eight pots a day.

Often – and especially during the summers when Bangalore experiences water shortages – these locked taps could not be operated, because shortages meant that paying neighbourhoods in Laggere could be deprived of their rights as paying consumers. Water provided in these locked taps was thus unreliable, as well as being inconvenient. The taps were opened for an hour each day, with at least 20–25 homes relying on a single tap, and during sum-mers, the access was often limited to twice a week. Due to the little water they were now able to access, women had to ensure additional water from other sources. Working women who were not available in the daytime to fetch water at erratic times could not rely on this supply, and they reported buying water from nearby middle-class homes at INR 5 per pot of water.

Apart from public taps, residents also accessed water illegally, connecting their homes to a water pipe close by, and covering the tap to ensure they were not found out. Many of these hidden connections were often in poor condition, with the possibility of water being contaminated by sand and gravel around these pipes. Because such illegal connections depend on the pressure of water in the pipes from which they are drawn, connections at certain points often did not work.

When water became very scarce and could not even be bought from middle-class homes in the neighbourhood, residents lobbied a councillor to pay for water trucks to supply the area. As Neela, one of the women I interviewed, told me:

> We had no problems for water earlier, there were three public taps and it was more than enough for all the 50 of us [families], as water was supplied for much longer. Even during the summers we would get water every day ... but now, we have to call the councillor for the truck every two days ... now if they [the middle-class neighbours] see us taking water, they call the water man and complain. (Interview, 4 January 2013)

Councillors often pay for this water at their own expense, with the hope of using this help to obtain votes in the next elections. Water is thus politically organised and the residents of Laggere have, despite the efforts of the BWSSB, been able to ensure free water most of the times, except for short periods when they may have to pay for water. After the 2002 decision of the BWSSB to reduce public taps, the councillor claimed that his expenditure on water trucks had gone up to more than twice the amount he spent earlier.

The implications for women and gender relations

Within households, women are responsible for ensuring adequate water for the household. During the six years of my research in the area, I saw a constant queue of women and girls, and rarely a few young boys, standing in the queues for water at borewells and public taps. These women and girls have to juggle their responsibilities for water collection, cleaning, washing, and laundry, with other responsibilities at home and outside. For women who are engaged in employment or income generation, Sundays are spent washing the family's clothes, and bathing themselves and their children. Sunday, far from being a holiday and a day of leisure, is to use the words of one of the garment factory workers:

> the hardest days of the week, when we have to complete all the work that has piled up during the week and in addition also sometimes host relatives or guests and cook special meals for the family. By the time I put my head down on the pillow, my body hurts.

The irregularity of access to water, and the need to find it from varied sources according to changes in availability and ability to pay, which fluctuates constantly, makes this already enormous workload even more difficult. The decreasing free water taps led to them spending between two and three hours each day attempting to patch together the water supplies they need for the home, including collecting water from middle-class homes in the neighbourhood. The lack of regular access to water also meant women bore the burden of hygiene, sanitation, and health within households.

Each home in the area relied on a woman at home to ensure access to water. As accessing water takes up a good amount of time each day, this work, in addition to other domestic work and care responsibilities, firmly situates women within the realm of their homes, reinforcing gendered roles in the process. Hence, water and the difficulties of obtaining it can prevent women from earning money. I asked Sushma, one of the residents, if she had considered working. She explained:

> Yes. I do want to [work]. But my work at home is just enough for me. Children need to go to school, and I also need to pack food for my husband … water is a real problem … at home, they will not send me anywhere [to work] … he says, why, I will look after everything, you keep quiet … . only if there is a water problem near the house, you look into it, is what he says. (Interview, 9 January 2013)

The fact that the new privatisation policies are resulting in increased time spent seeking water is particularly striking given that a key argument supporting the idea of privatisation is that paid connections take away the drudgery of lining up in queues, and will result in a lot of time saved, that women can then use to generate income for their households. However, this is only for those households who can afford piped water into their houses; the potential of privatisation and piped connections is clearly absent for the women in poverty whose access to public water supplies was never good, but is further constrained and challenged by policies that discriminate against the poorest in society.

Of the 47 women I interviewed, 20 women were employed, and the others were primarily responsible for the care of children or others in the family and shouldered the domestic responsibility solely. Of these 20, nine women spoke of having to give up jobs as domestic maids due to the increasing amount of time spent on collecting water. All these women thus had to rely on male earnings, and saw a dip in their household incomes.

When male earnings increase and the family is able to take care of its needs, women are increasingly motivated to quit work and manage their homes. My observation was that upper middle-class norms of housewifery were imitated and aspired to amongst the urban poor as it signifies a certain class status that is represented through the control of women.[8]

Sushma, above, recounted that she was 'allowed' to work when the family had a loan to pay. More accurately, the need to pay the loan created a crisis for the household and she was needed to work to help support the family, even though she had an increasing burden of supplying water for the home.

A majority of the women I interviewed (27 out of 47) were unemployed and were most often primarily responsible for all domestic work, and were also sometimes responsible for the care of children or aged family members. Apart from these responsibilities, a number of women had restricted mobility, due to patriarchal norms that rejected any possibility of women working. In contexts like Laggere, a mathematical conversion of time savings into income generation does not reflect the realities of different kinds of paid and unpaid women's work: either its value or its availability. Even if women are able and willing to be gainfully employed, these decisions still depend on the availability of jobs or other income-generating opportunities.

The poor pay most for water

A particularly shocking finding was that the residents of Laggere were paying much more for water compared to their upper-class counterparts during times of water crisis, such as during summers. This echoes the findings mentioned above from earlier research (Prahalad and Hammond 2002). However, my research shows that over longer periods of time, the urban poor do pay less than the other classes, because of the provision of free water which contributes to reducing the costs they incur.

Of the 47 women I interviewed, 33 women spoke of spending between INR 100 and 150 per month for drinking water alone, buying pots of water at INR 5 and 10 each from neighbouring middle-class homes, and the remaining 17 women spoke of spending between INR 150 and 200 per month. Importantly, however, these payments were not regular, and rose during periods of water crisis. The practice of patching together the required water supply from various sources meant expenditure on water varied. Wherever possible, savings were made through using ground water to wash clothes, and using illegal connections. Potable water was reserved for drinking and cooking, so the amount of water they purchase was limited. There are periods of time when their expenditure on water is nil or very little and at certain other times, such as during summers, it is much higher than what the middle class pay.

Over the period of five years during which I conducted my research, of the 50 women I interviewed, the large majority remained sceptical about paid water, and did not want to submit to monthly payments. Those who preferred paid connections were better off, with the large majority consisting of dual-income households. In such households where there is more disposable income combined with less time to fetch and store water, women prefer paid water connections. The assumption that the urban poor can afford to and are willing to pay more for water is thus flawed on two counts: first, it does not consider class differences amongst the urban poor and, secondly, it does not account for the fluctuating costs borne by the poor for water over long periods of time.

For much of the urban poor women I interviewed, the issue of water aroused a lot of heated debate and discussion. Three better-off women spoke of wanting paid connections, but all others – 47 out of the 50 involved in my research – thought of free water as a right, something they are entitled to. The vast majority of the other women I interacted with in focus group discussions, conversations, and other interactions, shared this understanding of water as an entitlement, and wanted free provision. Women are thus not passive victims, but active agents resisting commodification by insisting on free water. As Kathleen O'Reilly (2006, 2008) shows in her work on water commodification in Rajasthan, women rely on their own experiences to inform their opinions and do not submit completely to what they are told.

Women felt their entitlement to water was particularly strong due to their poverty. One of the respondents, Anita, responded to me when I suggested that the group she was part of could mobilise the KSBD to obtain water connections for them:

> But why should we pay, we earn very little, we live in these small homes ... you can see we can hardly stretch our feet without touching the walls ... How can we pay when we have no money to pay ... the government should give us water ... we need it to live ... it's our right ... how can they take it and sell it to us? Do we pay to breathe the air ... water is like air, it belongs to us all. (Anita, interview, 23 June 2015)

Women thus continue to see water – and claim it – as a public good, something they have a right to, by virtue of having life, and by virtue of their poverty. This response needs to be contextualised within a long history of water provision that acknowledged their human right to water, by providing the poor with public taps.

Resisting commoditisation: strategies to obtain free water

The fact that people had left a slum to come to live in the Laggere area for 'rehabilitation' meant little, because the area had no access to services such as water, so little had improved in their material realities. The urban poor who earlier relied on political trade-offs to secure access to free water in the slums they had left, continue to do so in their rehabilitation homes. As shown earlier, women are often forced to pay for water, purchasing this from middle-class neighbours. But they are also actively opposing the principle of privatisation by using their existing social relationships to help them secure water.

As discussed earlier, the municipal councillors negotiate access through public taps, by calling the water man[9] and ensuring that water is supplied through the locked public taps in the area. Councillors with a good track record of serving the poor often see themselves re-elected and this motivates them to continue serving the poor. They view their work enabling access to free water as an essential democratic role and not as an act of 'illegal access' or theft of water as the BWSSB terms it (BWSSB 2016). One councillor in Laggere explained how he organised water supply for the urban poor in his ward through representatives of the urban poor – referred to as leaders:

> After the construction [of the rehabilitation housing], the Slum Board does not even put a tap or sanitation or anything for that matter ... They [the leaders] are personally present at the water points, identify where there is no water and get water tankers to those spots. They switch on the borewells and give them ten pots of water ... Our ward needs to get a good name and we want development in our ward. Our leaders have got us votes by campaigning for us door to door. This ward has given 90 per cent of the votes to me. We need to also give 90 per cent to them, right?[10]

Over and above their official duties, municipal councillors see value in sometimes personally paying for water to ensure their re-election. If water is supplied and the residents of Laggere are pleased, this translates into votes, while councillors who do not carry out their promises are voted out. These arrangements are not formally approved by the BWSSB. While the BWSSB institutionally adopts a stance against free water, in practice officials of the BWSSB in charge of releasing water work closely with the municipal councillor to enable access to free water to the urban poor. Because many of these water men also come from the economically lower classes, they frequently sympathise with the urban poor and enable free water in stealth, without drawing the attention of those who can put a stop to it – such as middle-class residents or senior officials at the BWSSB.[11]

This relationship between the urban poor and elected representatives has been described in urban studies literature in opposing terms. On the one hand, it is seen as inclusive governance (Benjamin and Bhuvaneshwari 2001; Benjamin 2000), or deep democracy (Appadurai 2001). On the other, it is described as clientelism (de Wit 1989) or patronage (de Wit and Berner 2009).

In my own earlier work, I have argued that these relations of dependence are mutual, and that the urban poor demand accountability through the exercise of their votes, holding accountable both elected representatives as well as their own leaders who are instrumental in determining the terms of exchange of votes for services (Haritas 2013). As Bharathi, one of the residents, explained to me:

> He can win only when thousands of people vote for him. He will eventually have to come here to ask for votes. We have come today to his house begging, but he also had come to our door step that day begging for votes. (Interview, 6 January 2012)

The right to water is thus enforced politically, and not through a recourse to law. Elected representatives are aware of the importance of water, specially in areas such as Laggere that has a dominant urban poor population, capable of influencing electoral outcomes. They are aware that their performance as representatives is closely linked to the supply of water. The ability of councillors to influence water men, even if they are unable to influence the decisions of the BWSSB, enables them to ensure urban poor access to water. In the process, urban poor women are able to bypass recent policy changes on water, reinstating free water supply through their everyday negotiations with the state.

Conclusion

As water transitions from a public resource that the state is responsible to provide for its citizens to a consumer good, the urban poor in Bangalore are witnessing a transformation in the manner in which their free access to water is viewed by the state. As earlier norms of providing free water to the poor through public stand posts are increasingly being replaced by initiatives to include the poor as paying customers, the urban poor women in my research resist these moves by laying claim to water as a basic need essential to life itself. They thus frame the issue of water as an issue of justice, asserting the need to uphold their human right to water.

Claiming free water is becoming increasingly difficult and increasing the burden on women. The commodification of water puts immense responsibility on women to ensure the health and hygiene of their families. As commodification results in lesser access to water, women have to fight harder for fewer pots of water, spend more time accessing water, and thus more time on domestic tasks. In the homes of the urban poor in Laggere, with increased time spent on accessing water, daughters and rarely sons are roped into helping their mothers, taking away time that could otherwise be spent on play, education, or leisure.

Privatisation of water does not address the realities of the urban poor and the class differences amongst them. Expecting them to adhere to a price that is set universally for all classes may have very negative consequences for women and girls – in particular, women and girls living in poverty – and gender relations. Women are resisting privatisation in a range of covert and overt ways – including using political connections – because they see the impossibility of paying for water, which is a basic need, and a human right.

Notes

1. In Chameli Singh v. State of UP (1996) 2 SCC 549: AIR 1996 SC 1051, the Supreme Court held 'That right to live guaranteed in any civilised society implies the right to food, water, decent environment, education, medical care and shelter. These are basic human rights known to any civilised society. All civil, political, social and cultural rights enshrined in the Universal Declaration on Human Rights and Convention or under the Constitution of India cannot be exercised without these basic human rights'. The Supreme Court has further held the primacy of drinking water over other

water uses, observing that 'Drinking is the most beneficial use of water and this need is so paramount that it cannot be made subservient to any other use of water, like irrigation so that right to use of water for domestic purpose would prevail over other needs' (Delhi Water Supply and Sewage Disposal Undertaking v. State of Haryana (1996) 2 SCC 572: AIR 1996 SC 2992).

2. On 15 December 2014, the High Court in Mumbai ruled that Mumbai's local authority, the Brihanmumbai Municipal Corporation, should come up with a policy to supply water to illegal slumdwellers, stating that the Right to Water is an integral part of the Right to Life under Chapter 21 of the Indian Constitution (Pani Haq Samiti v. Brihan Mumbai Municipal Corporation and Others, 2012).

3. UN Water Decade Programme on Advocacy & Communication, Information Brief on Implementing Water Resource Management, see www.un.org/waterforlifedecade/waterandsustainabledevelopment2015/images/implementing_water_eng.pdf (last checked 31 May 2017).

4. Report submitted by the subject group on infrastructure, in April 2000: http://indiaimage.nic.in/pmcouncils/reports/; report on urban water and sanitation: http://indiaimage.nic.in/pmcouncils/reports/infra/ichap8.htm (last checked 31 May 2017).

5. Water is being commercialised through market-based reforms in Bangalore, moving away from reliance on public investment in the water sector to financing by users, municipal bonds, and other forms of debt. As Ranganathan *et al.* (2009) point out, this commercialisation entails institutional and financial changes in the management of water.

6. Poor settlements are often located on land that they do not own and is thus considered to be illegally occupied. Legal titles are required to obtain piped water supply from the BWSSB and since the poor cannot provide legal titles to the land they occupy, they are unable to obtain piped connections. In the case of slum rehabilitation areas, where my research was conducted, the slum board allots homes but retains ownership. Here again, those living in it do not possess ownership documents required to obtain a piped connection.

7. The BWSSB was set up in 1964 and was responsible for water infrastructure, operation, and maintenance, operating independent of the state government. The BWSSB took responsibility for ensuring an adequate water supply; the creation of sewerage network and safe disposal of sewage; preparation and implementation of plans and schemes for augmenting water supplies; safe disposal of sewage; and the levy and collection of water charges on a 'no loss no profit basis', aiming to ensure a sustainable system. However, the vision and mission of the BWSSB is focused on water quality and customer satisfaction, rather than ensuring access to water. For further information, see https://bwssb.gov.in/content/vision-mission (last checked 28 February 2017).

8. In my research, women in most better-off households were often stopped or prevented from working outside the home. A higher income and a relatively higher-class status also accompanies middle-class values that emphasise the role of the woman at home. This idea of the middle-class domestic housewife is a product of colonial relations in which

Indian womanhood was constructed in stark opposition to the British memsahib – with the modern Indian woman embodying both education and cultural refinement, without forsaking her place at home and her role of caregiver (Chatterjee 1989).

9. The 'water man' is an official of the BWSSB who is responsible for releasing water through the pipelines serving different areas. The term 'water man' or 'valve man' is commonly used to refer to these officials.

10. In this particular ward in Laggere where this councillor was elected, the dominant population resides in rehabilitation housing, while the situation differs in wards with an equal or lower share of urban poor population.

11. Benjamin and Bhuvaneshwari (2001), in their work on urban poor and governance in Bangalore, describe this as inclusive governance in which a 'politics of stealth' is used strategically by urban poor groups to claim resources. They define the politics of stealth as the importance for poor groups and their alliances to operate in a low-key, strategic, and 'non-visible' way, allowing them to subvert competing claims on resources and location. While they specifically focus on urban poor claims on land, this argument of 'stealth' also applies to the manner in which the urban poor access free water. In my research, I found that a complaint by a middle-class resident of an adjoining neighbourhood or a senior official at the BWSSB could well bring the free water supply to a halt. Thus, water is often provided erratically at different points of time during the day for a short period of time, stealthily enabling access, without drawing the attention of those who might complain.

Acknowledgements

I thank the hospitality and support of the women and men from the slum rehabilitation area of Laggere whose voices inform this chapter. All names provided here are changed to ensure anonymity. I thank Caroline Sweetman for the meticulous editing and her comments and suggestions that have vastly improved this chapter. I also thank Dr. Vinod Vyasulu, Vice Dean, Jindal School of Government and Public Policy, O.P.Jindal Global University, Haryana for his comments and inputs into this chapter. Most importantly I thank Professor Christine Verschuur and Professor Isabelle Milbert, Graduate Institute of International and Development Studies for their guidance and the Swiss National Science Foundation for its generous PhD grant that allowed me to conduct this ethnographic research in the best conditions possible. I also thank Professor Sundar Sarukkai, National Institute of Advanced Studies, Bangalore for his support to conduct a last phase of research in 2015. I thank Professor Supriya Roy Chowdhury, Institute for Social and Economic Change, Bangalore for her kind support.

Notes on contributor

Kaveri Thara is the pen name of Kaveri Ishwar Haritas, Assistant Professor, Jindal School of Government and Public Policy, O.P.Jindal Global University, Haryana. Email: kiharitas@gmail.com

References

Appadurai, Arjun (2001) 'Deep democracy: urban governmentality and the horizon of politics', *Environment and Urbanization* 13(2): 23–43

Benjamin, Solomon (2000) 'Governance, economic settings and poverty in Bangalore', *Environment and Urbanization* 12(1): 35–56

Benjamin, Solomon and R. Bhuvaneshwari (2001) 'Democracy, Inclusive Governance and Poverty in Bangalore', IDD Working Paper, no. 26, Birmingham: International Development Department, University of Birmingham International Development Department, Birmingham

BWSSB (2016) 'Services for Urban Poor'. http://bwssb.gov.in/bwssbuat/content/services-0 (last checked 6 June 2017)

Chatterjee, Partha (1989) 'Colonialism, nationalism, and colonialized women: the contest in India', *American Ethnologist* 16(4): 622–33

Connors, Genevieve (2005) 'When utilities muddle through: pro-poor governance in Bangalore's public water sector', *Environment & Urbanization* 17(1): 201–18

Connors, Geneviève and Clarissa Brocklehurst (2006) 'A Utility's Pro-Poor Approach in Bangalore', New Delhi: Water and Sanitation Program South Asia

de Wit, Joop (1989) 'Clientelism, competition and poverty: the ineffectiveness of local organizations in a Madras Slum', in Frans Schuurman and Ton Van Naerssen (eds.) *Urban Social Movements in the Third World*, London: Routledge, 63–90

de Wit, Joop and Erhard Berner (2009) 'Progressive patronage? municipalities, NGOs, CBOs and the limits to Slum Dwellers' empowerment', *Development and Change* 40(5): 927–47

Express News Service (2011) 'Houses Razed in Jayabheema Nagar.'

Government of India (2005) *Jawaharlal Nehru National Urban Renewal Mission: Overview*, http://jnnurm.nic.in/wp-content/uploads/2011/01/UIGOverview.pdf (last checked 6 June 2017)

Government of Karnataka (2003) 'Karnataka Urban Drinking Water and Sanitation Policy, 2003'. http://www.siudmysore.gov.in/pdf/reading material/W&WWM/RM.pdf (last checked 6 June 2017)

Haritas, Kaveri (2013) 'Gender identity in urban poor mobilizations: evidence from Bengaluru', *Environment and Urbanization* 25(1): 125–38, doi:10.1177/0956247813477811

Karnataka Slum Development Board (2016) 'Slum Details at a Glance', Karnataka Government, http://www.karnataka.gov.in/ksdb/Pages/Slum-Statistics.aspx (last checked 6 June 2017)

Lele, S., V. Srinivasan, P. Jamwal, B.K. Thomas, M. Eswar, and T. Md. Zuhail (2013) Water Management in Arkavathy Basin: A Situation Analysis. Environment and Development Discussion Paper No. 1, Bengaluru, Karnataka: ATREE

Menezes, Naveen (2015) 'BWSSB Moves Ahead with Cauvery Fifth Stage Work', *Deccan Herald*, http://www.deccanherald.com/content/513447/bwssb-moves-ahead-cauvery-fifth.html# (last checked 6 June 2017)

Menon, Parvathi (2001) 'Cautious Corporatisation', *Frontline*, 18(13) Jun 23-Jul 06, http://www.frontline.in/static/html/fl1813/18130880.ht (last checked 6 June 2017)

O'Reilly, Kathleen (2006) '"Traditional" women, "modern" water: Linking gender and commodification in Rajasthan, India', Geoforum 37(6): 958–72, doi:10.1016/j.geoforum.2006.05.008

O'Reilly, Kathleen (2008) 'Insider/Outsider Politics: Implementing Gendered Participation in Water Resource Management', in Bernadette P. Resurrección and Rebecca Elmhirst, *Gender and Natural Resource Management: Livelihoods, Mobility and Interventions*, London and New York: Earthscan, 195–212

Piper, Karen (2015) *The Price of Thirst: Global Water Inequality and the Coming Chaos*, Minneapolis and London: University of Minnesota Press

Prahalad, C.K. and Allen Hammond (2002) 'Serving the World's Poor, Profitably', *Harvard Business Review*, September, 48–57

Ranganathan, Malini, Lalitha Kamath and Vinay Baindur (2009) 'Piped water supply to greater Bangalore: putting the cart before the horse?', *Economic & Political Weekly* XLIV(33): 53–62

Rao, Mohit M. (2016) 'City Fails to Keep up with Rise in Slums', *The Hindu*, 29 January

Wadhawan, Anup and Geeta Sharma (2007) 'Engaging with Citizens to Improve Services', New Delhi: Water and Sanitation Program South Asia

CHAPTER 8

Domesticating water supplies through rainwater harvesting in Mumbai

Cat Button

Abstract

Mumbai is a city where 60 per cent of the population are living in poverty in informal settlements, with low – and decreasing – water access, and low resilience to water shortage. In the middle-class areas of the city, inhabitants are being made responsible for securing their own water supplies via rainwater-harvesting technology, which is increasingly installed in new housing. This shifts responsibility for water provision from city authorities to private households. The domestication of water supplies could potentially give residents more control, and could also change the gendered power balance of water provision. However, this chapter argues that making the middle classes responsible for their own water provision in a context of water shortage and environmental concerns has justice implications. People living in poverty are not able to self-provision in this way; yet on the other hand, the move could free up more of the piped water supply. The chapter draws on three case studies offering different experiences of the impact of the policy, to reflect on concepts of power, gender, and environmental justice.

Keywords: Water; infrastructure; domestic; Mumbai; governance; rainwater harvesting

Introduction

In the city of Mumbai, India, 60 per cent of the population are living in poverty in informal settlements, with low – and decreasing – water access, and low resilience to water shortage (Srivastava and Echanove 2014). The city authorities have struggled to provide water to residents in the past (Gandy 2006). In a context of low and decreasing water access and low resilience to water shortages, innovative ways of solving the shortage are needed, and, '[f]or the first time in its history, the city's municipal corporation and its water engineers have been engaged in educational and outreach programmes to encourage changes in household water use and the introduction of water-saving technologies' (Gandy 2006, 19).

As part of this agenda, the responsibility for securing water resources in Mumbai's middle-class households has been shifted on to the residents

http://dx.doi.org/10.3362/9781788530866.008

themselves, via rainwaterharvesting technologies installed for individual households. In Mumbai's domestic properties, decentralised water provision by the general population of an area (from bore-wells and tankers) is being extended or replaced by rainwater harvesting. This means that more water is being supplied at the level of an individual building, and therefore housing is becoming a site of production, not just consumption. This blurring of the boundaries between supplier and consumer, and between housing and infrastructure, has implications for the governance of infrastructure and distribution of power (see Bakker 2010).

The case studies featured here are the result of fieldwork during two extended periods in Mumbai (between 2009 and 2011), and several subsequent trips to India. Each of the three focuses on rainwater-harvesting systems and how they are used. The first concerns a middle-class apartment building that was an early adopter of environmental decentralised infrastructure; the second is another apartment building with rainwater harvesting where residents reflect on the experiences of the female maids who work there but live in an informal settlement; and the third is a slum that has a rainwater-harvesting system for a toilet block.

In this study, I was keen to include a variety of methods such as using photographs, walking interviews during visits to buildings, and ethnographic observations. I developed photographic methodologies around these visits, which were particularly useful to the investigations. This included in-depth site visits to 22 apartment buildings in north Mumbai, and one informal settlement.

The focus on the middle classes and professionals brought interviews to prominence as a key method to collect data to address all research questions. Interviews of individuals or small groups lasted between 15 minutes and two hours, with an average of about half an hour. Most of those interviewed were professionals or experts (architects, consultants, property developers, non-government organisation officers, government officials, etc.; 24 male and nine female), interviewed in their own offices in Mumbai. I also interviewed residents (seven male and nine female) and servants (one male and two female). I interviewed one watchman (Mumbai, 12 February 2011) and two maids (Mumbai, 8 February 2011). The watchman gave me insights into how the building had changed over the past decade and the maids explained some of the everyday practices they undertook.

Employers were often unwilling to let me speak to servants because they did not consider the servants' knowledge important. One building secretary could not grasp (after a year of explaining) why I would want to talk to staff when he could explain everything and he thought watchman would not know anything (interviews, Mumbai, 2009–2011). I repeatedly met with this rhetoric of servants not knowing anything and their input to my research not being needed. This dismissal of needing to speak to other people also brought out the power dynamics of knowledge and justice issues arising from assumed superiority of some respondents. I was keen to speak to servants who used water that was harvested, so that I could understand exactly what they did, whether practices had changed since installation, and what their knowledge of the systems was. However, there were language barriers in speaking to them, leaving me with no option but to use a 'gatekeeper', who was often also their employer, as translator. This compromised results as servants might have adapted their answers to please their employers. It also meant that I was not hearing their 'true voice' and something may have been altered or omitted in translation. I was also able to use my observations from site visits and ethnographic methods to investigate these everyday practices. My primary data are also supported by policy and media sources, and attending conferences was also a useful way to gain an insight into official standpoints of organisations and government departments.

This chapter begins with an introduction to Mumbai's water supplies, followed by a discussion of rainwater harvesting as a technology. I then move on to focus on domestication, a concept that I used to gain a rounded understanding of the impact and implications of rainwater harvesting for environmental sustainability, the satisfaction of water, sanitation, and hygiene (WASH) needs, and power relations: between individual households and the city governance, between middle-class and poorer residents of Jaipur, and between women and men. The three case studies are then analysed. Issues of power and justice are drawn out in the discussion, and this leads to conclusions and recommendations.

Mumbai's water infrastructure

Water infrastructure is highly differentiated and uneven across Mumbai. The Municipal Corporation of Greater Mumbai (MCGM, also known as BMC) still bears the sole responsibility for water supply in the city (BrihanMumbai Municipal Corporation 2003). However, in reality the municipality is just one of the actors in a system of governing (Bulkeley and Betsill 2003). This is evident in the provision of tankers by private enterprises and the 'water mafia' to fill demand. The MCGM acknowledges that there is a shortfall in this supply, and this has led the municipality to implement water-saving tactics, and to shift responsibility. This is instead of other routes such as investing on the current system to remove leakages or selling of the (lucrative) water utility for privatisation.

> It is expected that there should be an active participation of the citizens in water conservation (saving). Citizens have to generate water for secondary requirements through rain water harvesting or recycling. (MCGM 2008, 1)

This approach to water-saving in the city of Mumbai might be seen as a positive move, but it is more complex than that. Underlying it is an attempt by the government to roll back its responsibility for water provision. The splintered provision of water in Mumbai has roots in the colonial planning of the city (Zérah 2008). The water department was created in 1860 to supply water from lakes when the existing wells and tanks were insufficient, due to drought and urbanisation, and yet the colonial government did not have aspirations that mains water would be universally provided (Anand 2011). Although the network of supply pipes has been extended, it has not kept up with urban growth, and a shortage of water supply has been created.

Mains drinking water comes from several reservoirs or lakes outside the city, but is only supplied for a few hours per day, to each area of the city (Sule no date). In middle-class housing, an illusion of constant supply is created through the storage of mains water in tanks to be used at other times in the day, and supplementation by other forms of access, such as tankers and bore-wells, for non-potable purposes (Button 2017). For poorer households, mains water connections are often from stand-pipes in the street, shared between several households, and water must be collected in buckets whenever the taps spring to life (Anand 2011; Graham *et al.* 2013). It is often women and girls who spend time collecting water and the rhythm of the stand pipe can re-order their days. Many other informal residents have no mains connection leading to a reliance on expensive water tankers or the creation of illegal connections to mains water pipes (*ibid.*).

Crises and failures of the system are often seen as moments in which the infrastructure of a city is suddenly foregrounded (Graham and Marvin 2001; Kaika 2005). Domestic water supply is therefore presented as operating in an isolated 'black box' in much of the literature from the global North, and only becomes visible when it breaks down (Graham 2006; Shove 2003). However, it could be argued that the everyday occurrence of inadequacy and failure of Mumbai's infrastructure keeps water supply visible as an issue. In Mumbai, shortages and failures are endemic. Frank Trentmann (2009) argues that disruption is normal in most systems (and not just in the global South); and argues that the reaction to these disruptions depends on the degree to which they are accepted as normal. In Mumbai, interruptions occur often, and the infrastructure is highly differentiated and flexible as a result. Those households that do have a piped mains water connection only receive water for a few hours per day and store it in tanks as well as using other forms of supply. Thus, water is brought into homes and domesticated in different ways.

The middle classes (and elites) have the financial means to secure their clean water supply, by calling for additional water tankers, digging borewells, and now through rainwater harvesting. The promotion of 'green' infrastructure (such as rainwater harvesting) is a new way of prioritising the systems for the wealthy, as those who can afford to fund additional sources can create their own water supply. Many of Mumbai's residents do not have access to formal water supplies, but self-funded decentralised supplies are now being emphasised as a solution to deficits in water infrastructure (McFarlane 2008b). The addition of rainwater-harvesting infrastructure to a building does not just help its residents, but improves water provision across the city by reducing demand, and is suggested as a solution to shortage by the municipality

(MCGM 2008). Rainwater harvesting and ground water recharge may also improve water quality from borewells, and reduce cracking and collapse of buildings (Sule no date). The increasing provision of alternative technologies at the scale of individual buildings should mean that less water (and electricity and municipal solid waste) infrastructure needs to be provided centrally by the state or private companies to meet everyone's demands.

The installation of these rainwater-harvesting technologies, however, amounts to an acceptance of the reduced supply by the state, and normalises water shortage. This might be accepted by the middle classes, who can increase their resilience to shortage by installing other water sources, but it could actually reduce the water access of the poorest residents by legitimising reduction in state water supplies for residential areas. Those people living in informal settlements are likely to be most adversely affected by the rolling back of state provision, rather than the extension of it, as well as being most vulnerable to water shortages. The management of water supplies and collection of water often adds to the double burden of women and girls in Mumbai.

Rainwater harvesting as a solution to water shortages

> Green buildings also need rainwater harvesting and water recycling. Green buildings reduce costs, not just for residents but also for city level. (Professor Saugata Roy, Minister of State for Urban Development, speaking at the National Conference on Green Design: Buildings and Habitats, New Delhi, 8 January 2011)

Globally, people are seeking solutions to water insecurity, and the harvesting of rainwater offers potential in many contexts. There are many different ways to collect rainwater depending on the circumstances. In many regions of the world, water is collected from roofs of buildings, and stored in tanks either above or below ground Handia *et al.* (2003) look at examples in urban Zambia and Kahinda *et al.* (2007) discuss rainwater harvesting in the context of rural South Africa. Villages in Northern India, where water is scarce due to low rainfall, have collected rainwater in large ponds or wells for use by the community for centuries, particularly for watering crops (Pandey *et al.* 2003). In contrast, in dense urban areas and monsoonal climates, like Mumbai, water systems that recharge the ground water or aquifers are favoured. In these contexts, if rainwater is collected, it is often used for specific practices, such as watering plants or flushing toilets, and this is made possible due to the fact that these two forms of water supply remain separate.

Rainwater harvesting offers a new source of water that could be transformative for Mumbai-dwellers with limited access to water, especially the urban poor. This substitution of water supplies can be framed as an environmental solution that could save water and alleviate stress on Mumbai's infrastructure, with the added benefit that the limited supplies from other sources are freed up to be used more abundantly for other practices. Rainwater harvesting has been compulsory since 2003 in newly constructed buildings in Mumbai, built on plots over 1,000 m² (BrihanMumbai Municipal Corporation 2003) and in those constructed on sites over 300 m² since 2007 (MCGM 2008). Retrofits are becoming increasingly popular also, as the municipality reduces mains water supplies and promotes water-saving initiatives, and this reduces reliance on mains water supplies.

In my research, a Municipal Officer working for MCGM stated:

> We made that it [rainwater harvesting] is compulsory for all new build-ings. But why only new buildings? Why not for the old buildings? … because I understand that would be a constraint of space. The new build-ings have a lot of space and they follow a lot of new rules and norms, which are very different from the older norms. But still you should allow anyone to do it and it should be compulsory for everyone. (Interview, Mumbai, 20 January 2011)

All three of the case studies in my research were of retrofits to existing domestic buildings. These are becoming popular through the incentives of water security and economic gains, rather than by legislation. The officer in charge of rainwater harvesting at the BMC told me that most of the requests for information are from residents of existing buildings looking to retrofit and take control of their water supplies, rather than developers constructing new apartment buildings (interview, Mumbai, 10 February 2011). Thus, retrofits seem to be set to become an important, but unregulated, part of the urban environmental responses that bring additional water supplies into homes.

Domestication as a concept to help understand water provision

In my exploration of rainwater harvesting in Mumbai, I drew on the idea of domestication. The concept of 'domestication' denotes the taming and re-scaling of infrastructure to fit into the home, and has been used by several academics to explain the relationship between nature, cities, and homes.

Maria Kaika (2004) uses domestication as part of her explanation of how nature is tamed and brought into the modern home. The idea of domesti-cation draws on concepts of political power, control over nature, and the creation of comfort in the home. In particular, Maria Kaika uses the idea to conceptualise how modern homes control and sort nature. She sees domesti-cation as bringing nature into the home and taming it (such as piped potable water), and also excluding unwanted natural elements (such as sewage or pollution).

A second view of domestication comes from Elizabeth Shove (2003). She writes about how the uptake and adoption of a new technology into the everyday practices of the home can be thought of as domestication, to create comfort. For Shove, domestication takes places when technology is 'adapted, incorporated and converted' (*ibid.*, 55), through everyday practices in the home. Elizabeth Shove goes on to argue that, although available technology shapes human practices, the way in which technology is brought into homes and used in accordance with residents' requirements also feeds back into and changes the socio-technical system of water supply.

The idea of domestication was also taken up by a third writer, Eric Swyngedouw (2004), who researched water provision in Guayaquil, Ecuador. He sees the ability to domesticate your water and bring it into the home as an expression of social power (Swyngedouw 2004). The privatisation of responsibility for water provision changes the social contract between individual households and the city authorities. Private housing becomes a site of resource provision and control. Domestication can therefore be seen as an extension of urbanisation and the commodification of water. I found his analysis useful when looking at the ways water infrastructure is being taken into Mumbai's middle-class homes, and the effects of this on water provision not only for these households, but for different categories and groups of people, and for power relations in the city.

In the context of my case studies, these ideas about domestication of water supplies into the home or community were useful. I focused on the domestication of technology (Shove 2003), water (Swyngedouw 2004), and nature (Kaika 2004) to consider what it means to domesticate environmental infrastructure through the use of rainwater harvesting in the apartments of Mumbai.

The resident as consumer and supplier

> In most of the cases, it's the residents. Whether they have implemented it or not, it is the residents that come forward. And especially it is one resident who is aware of it and then they build up momentum in their society. And then usually we have done, I don't know how many presentations to residential housing societies. We go there and show them what is rainwater harvesting and why and how it will benefit them. (Architect and scholar, interview, Mumbai, 13 February 2010)

Residential buildings are an important scale at which to investigate environmental technologies and governance. Housing brings together services, both through large-scale centralised infrastructures and small-scale decentralised systems, for use in a variety of practices.

Apartment Building 1: early adopters

The first of my three case studies focused on a middle-class apartment building in the northern suburbs of Mumbai. Rainwater harvesting was retrofitted several years before my visit, and was a great success. The building's co-operative secretary was engaged in raising awareness of the technology in Mumbai. They had also subsequently installed a solar water heater and photovoltaic cells to power lighting in communal areas.

Economic reasons were cited by residents for the installation of rainwater harvesting, especially in buildings that were previously relying heavily on tankers to reinforce their water supply. The capital costs may be high, but the savings quickly add up. The male resident and secretary of the co-operative society at Apartment Building 1 told me:

> People take these environmental technologies as a cost, but it is not a cost. It's an investment. (Interview, Mumbai, 9 January 2010)

The use of rainwater as a source of potable water is a controversial issue. Although rain can be one of the purest sources of water, the methods of collection, storage, and treatment are vital to maintaining the quality. With the correct storage and/or treatment there is no reason why harvested rainwater cannot be used for all purposes (Handia *et al.* 2003). However, although the rainwater is likely to be cleaner and safer than some of the sources in Mumbai, it was not seen as acceptable for use as potable water by the middle classes in this particular building. The same informant told me:

> One is the suspended matter is higher. The content of suspended matter, it comes from there. The second is that the bacteria count is a little higher. (Interview, 24 January 2011)

Harvested rainwater may still be used as potable water in extreme circumstances, and/or when a special filter is in place. At Apartment Building 1 they had a series of filters, including an ultraviolet filter, in place to supply potable water in times of extreme water shortage.

Following on from the success of providing their own water supply, some residents are looking to supply other services in their own buildings. This domestication of services sees buildings and homes becoming both the producers and consumers of resources: the ultimate in privatisation. Several buildings in Mumbai now have solar-water heating and/or photovoltaic panels to supply some of the residents' energy needs. In effect, they have begun to run their own private energy companies to govern their own resource supply. This changes the boundaries and relationships between the home, the buildings, and the city, and there is a shift in power dynamics alongside this growing resilience and resource security.

Apartment Building 2: learning from example and thinking about power relations between servants and employers

The residents of Apartment Building 2 were advised to adopt rainwater harvesting by the residents of Apartment Building 1. In addition to showing learning by example, I will focus on them here to discuss the issues of power and class relations that came up in the research as participants reflected on the issues around water supplies faced by their domestic servants.

The gardens at Apartment Building 2 showed the difference that harvesting rainwater can make. A female resident and head of household explained how the retrofitted rainwater-harvesting system has affected consumption and gardening practices. A woman resident of Apartment Building 2 stated:

> Where I used to tell the gardener – 'please, today don't water, water only once in three days, or once in five days'– now he does it merrily every day and he's happy. (Interview, Mumbai, 24 January 2011)

In the 11 months between two visits to Apartment Building 2, the gardens at this property became visibly more extensive and verdant. This greenery has the added benefit of cooling the microclimate around the building, making it more pleasant in a hot, humid area like Mumbai. Site visit observations confirmed that it is male servants who perform the watering of the gardens, either a dedicated gardener in large buildings and townships, or as an extra responsibility of the watchman as observed in smaller apartment buildings.

The number and extent of servant employment in India is high, and hiring servants can be used as proof of middle-class status and provide the convenience and lifestyle desired (Qayum and Ray 2011). This outsourcing of care work within the household means that it may be the servants who are most aware and in control of resources, and they could be more aware of environmental impacts on water supply in their own home lives.

> The labour is so cheap you get used to all this, you know, it's so comfortable. We have a couple of people working at home and everything is just set the way you want it and you don't have to do anything. (Property Developer, interview, Mumbai, 16 December 2009)

In Mumbai many of these servants live in informal settlements, with limited access to water and sanitation (Gandy 2008; McFarlane 2008a). Severe water shortages are impacting on life in these settlements, and middle-class residents are aware of this, and the fact that the resources and amenities they take for granted are not available where their servants live. The same woman resident quoted above described the problems that her maids report from the slums in which they live:

> All our maids come from there [a nearby slum], and they are always complaining. Last three days they just didn't have any water. Like they just had water for barely two hours and they just had a queue for one tap and a whole lot of … so she said 'all that we managed to gather was drinking water' so it's just no bathing, no other. Just bare essentials. So it is a huge problem. (Interview, Mumbai, 24 January 2011)

Some of the male servants may reside underneath the apartment building, in-between the cars parked in the raised plinth or in the stairwells but again have very different access to water.

This analysis has obvious gendered implications since women are the primary consumers and users of water in their role as family carers, and this division of labour is reflected in the gendered roles of servants. The female domestic workers contracted to perform care work are tasked with ensuring their employers have a ready supply of water in their homes. Gender therefore intersects with class.

Rainwater harvesting did have a measure of positive impact on servants' lives. Firstly, servants have access to clean water at work, even when there is a water shortage at home, and they may be able to access this for personal use. Water shortages at home are rarely reflected in a maid's work, but demonstrate the gendered nature of water practices and of the space of the home. Secondly, rainwater supplies may actually reduce the drudgery of collecting water from municipal supplies or supervising tanker deliveries, when middleclass homes experience water shortages:

> we use this water for 24 hours for flushing and all. Floor washing. We can get more water. 24 hours. (Male resident of a middle-class apartment building in Bandra West, interview, Mumbai, 24 January 2011)

Thirdly, rainwater can be used for a variety of tasks that are easier with plentiful water. Floors are washed by maids and cars are cleaned by watchmen every day, due to the very dusty conditions in Mumbai. Availability of additional water can make it easier to perform cleaning tasks. These are normalised practices that can increase water consumption (Shove 2003). However, the practice of floor washing can be carried out using a small amount of water.

> I use two buckets of water to clean the floors in the entire apartment. (Daily maid, interview, Mumbai, 8 February 2011)

In that building, rainwater is used for cleaning inside the homes, particularly the floors, and for cleaning the offices of the co-operative management; thus, reducing consumption of the mains water supply by changing sources, rather than practices. The power to choose the source and supply of drinking water and to ensure the quality of water for your family is a privilege not open to everyone (Gandy 2006). The everyday water practices using rainwater harvesting illustrate the power dynamics of the Indian middle-class home. They highlight the injustices of water provision by who performs a specific task and who has access to which water sources for their personal use, as shown by the reluctance of middle classes to consume rainwater, but allowing servants to do so. Despite middle-class fears about using rainwater as potable water, there was evidence of the water being made available for servants to drink and cook with: an example of how power relations are seen in play – and reinforced – through obvious differentiation around resource use. This also reveals some of the justice implications of water practices.

Informal settlement: domesticating the slum and the water supply

My third example here concerns the use of a rainwater-harvesting system in an informal settlement to flush the toilets of a communal toilet block.

I discovered only one rainwater-harvesting system in an informal settlement, and conducted interviews and made observations there. The rainwater-harvesting scheme is at an informal settlement in north Mumbai and was undertaken by a community-based organisation called Triratna Prerana Mandal (TPM) (Alfred Herrhausen Gesellschaft no date). Rainwater is collected from the outdoor play area and the roof of the community centre that TPM constructed. This water is now used to flush the public toilets at the centre. This shows the potential for much-needed rainwater-harvesting schemes in informal settlements, but there may not be space. TPM was also considering installing photovoltaic panels to power lighting and computers. This leads to the domestication of shared space; as everyday practices are undertaken at the community centre, it becomes part of people's homes.

The residents in the first and second examples, above, were able to secure their water services in the wider context of a secure lifestyle, but poorer citizens do not have the capacity to do this by retrofitting rainwater-harvesting systems. One major issue is space: the roofs and grounds are not individually large enough to collect rainwater for use by the residents. Space is also needed for storage or recharge into an aquifer or well. Rainwater harvesting can save recurring expenditure on water, but it requires an investment of capital. In addition, lack of security of tenure in informal settlements reduces the commitment to improvements. The MCGM favours redevelopment and rehabilitation, rather than upgrading and investment, in informal settlements.

There is also the issue of funding schemes and of political will. In Mumbai, the municipality is reluctant to supply informal settlements with infrastructure as this could legitimise the area (Graham *et al*. 2013). Decentralised systems could help bridge the infrastructure deficit, but the current focus for the city authorities is, rather, on promoting middle-class responses that are self-funded (Button 2017). Rainwater harvesting as a solution for middle classes normalises uneven water distribution. Lack of pressure from the middle classes to supply water lets the state 'off the hook', allowing it to roll back provision, and abandon aspirations for equitable water provision for all citizens of Mumbai.

Beyond privatisation

Privatisation of water is contested politically and the privatisation of water supplies has been undertaken across the world to varying degrees and in different ways. In India, the water supply has not been privatised in a formal way, leaving the ultimate responsibility for water provision to the state. However, in practice, some parts of water supply have been taken on by private endeavours; either for profit – as in the example of the water tankers of the 'Water Mafia'[1] – or to build personal resilience to fluctuations in supply, as in the example of the rainwater harvesting discussed in this paper, blurring state and non-state boundaries (Bulkeley and Schroeder 2011).

The rolling back of mains water supply by the municipality and the encouragement to save water and install rainwater-harvesting technology has led individual citizens to govern their own water supplies. This shifts governance debates from the interactions of institutions, to a focus on individuals within buildings. Residents now have more control over their water supplies, leading to more water availability at lower costs.

It could be suggested that this governing and supply of water, and other services, at the building level by private householders could reduce the amount of corruption experienced around water supply. Decentralisation and involvement of stakeholders in governance of resources, including water, has been seen to achieve this in other Indian states where moving from regional to local government water governance had increased corruption levels (Asthana 2008). However, the current situation in Mumbai could be characterised, using Karen Bakker's (2010) ideas, as going 'beyond privatisation' of water supply, in the sense of the residents and civil society taking responsibility for securing water supplies. When the state fails to provide services, some residents fill the gaps in provision by other means, such as harvesting rainwater to deal with water shortages.

Active interaction between providers and users of environmental services is important, and good links can lead to accountability in decision-making (Baud and Dhanalakshmi 2007). But what happens when the providers and users of those environmental services are the same people and places? In the case of Mumbai, privatisation of water supply through rainwater harvesting has occurred at the scale of the individual building, making suppliers and consumers the same actors. This domestication gives residents greater control over their supply through this extreme form of privatisation down to the micro/building scale. The governed and the governors have, in effect, become one and the same as the water supplies are domesticated.

Decentralised systems could help bridge the infrastructure deficit by freeing-up more of the municipal mains supply for use by other citizens. However, the potential to save municipal supplies for those who cannot afford rainwater systems does not appear to be realised; lack of a shared interest in saving water means some middle-class residents opt to use rainwater-harvesting systems and water-saving technology for uses deemed by them to be essential, but which people in poverty would not recognise as such. The availability of rainwater through harvesting has been found to increase water consumption of middle-class residents who can now afford to use water for other practices that were restricted before (such as watering gardens and washing cars frequently) (Button 2014).

Linking development commitments to providing water to all with the realities of today's rapidly growing cities in global South contexts involves adopting pragmatic and efficient solutions. It should not matter whether infrastructure consists of monolithic centralised systems or dispersed decentralised systems, as long as it is well-built, well-maintained, and provides resources to all citizens. Rainwater harvesting could be a solution if education and funding streams made it a technology available to all, and this will be a great missed opportunity if it continues to only be accessible to the middle classes.

Conclusions: domesticating infrastructure governance

There is an important difference between more people getting access to some water, and some people getting access to more water. The domestication of water supplies has produced middle classes that are becoming increasingly resilient to water (and energy) shortage and to some aspects of climate change. Yet the rolling back of state responsibility for water supply and promotion of middle-class responses to resource shortage has several consequences for the future of services in Mumbai.

It shifts the responsibility for governing water resources to the residents, reconfiguring their role to become both consumer and supplier. Housing is being re-cast as a provider of services, primarily of water through rainwater-harvesting interventions. The state is reinforcing this domestication, with middle-class residents as producers and consumers of decentralised 'green' resources, through rainwater-harvesting legislation and other initiatives.

Yet as I have argued, this domestication of water supplies, and their governance, is allowing the state to redefine its role as service provider, and roll back its responsibility for universal provision. My research suggests that the middle-class residents of Mumbai are potentially gaining more control, in contrast to more negative implications for the domestic workers whom they employ, and for the poorer residents of the city who are not able to afford rainwater-harvesting technologies.

The prioritisation of rainwater harvesting as a response to both shortage and to the environmental issues facing Mumbai is putting the needs and wants of the middle classes before those of the poor majority, who cannot afford to install a rainwater-harvesting system. Private middle-class residents are working to secure their water and energy supplies by retrofitting rainwater-harvesting systems. This decentralisation of resources redefines residential buildings' relationship with the city and the boundaries of infrastructure, and gives residents more power over their water. Yet this particular form of decentralisation of water provision has class and gendered implications, creating particular issues for informal slum-dwellers, and servants in their roles as paid domestic carers for their employers. Women have gendered responsibility for water use in domestic settings and are the least likely to participate in decision-making on water supply and infrastructure design, maintenance, and use.

In conclusion, this emphasis on middle-class responses to water shortage and environmental concerns has justice implications in a city where 60 per cent of the population live in informal settlements with reduced water access, and lower resilience. Because the middle classes are able to evolve ways of coping with the shortage of municipal water supplies, they accept the roll-back of state provision. As the middle classes collect and supply their own water they form a new type of localised privatisation, which feeds back into legislation and shifts power, governances, and changes the relationship with the city.

Note

1. The Water Mafia is a collection of people and organisations who control the black market in water. They make money by selling water illegally and accepting bribes. They are also known to use intimidation methods to secure their market (see Graham *et al.* 2013).

Notes on contributor

Cat Button is Senior Lecturer of Global Urbanisms in the School of Architecture Planning and Landscape at Newcastle University, UK. She is the degree programme director of MSc Urban Planning. Her interdisciplinary and international research focuses on how people and communities cope with having too little (or too much) water. Email: cat.button@ncl.ac.uk

References

Alfred Herrhausen Gesellschaft (no date) 'Deutsche Bank Urban Age Award 2007', https://www.alfredherrhausen-gesellschaft.de/en/urban-age/urban-age-award-2014.htm#tab_2007-br-mumbai (last checked 19 June 2017)

Anand, Nikhil (2011) 'PRESSURE: the PoliTechnics of water supply in Mumbai', *Cultural Anthropology* 26(4): 542–64

Asthana, Anand N. (2008) 'Decentalisation and corruption: evidence from drinking water sector', *Public Administration and Development* 28(3): 181–9

Bakker, Karen (2010) *Privatizing Water: Governance Failure and the World's Urban Water Crisis*, New York: Cornell University Press

Baud, Isa and R. Dhanalakshmi (2007) 'Governance in urban environmental management: comparing accountability and performance in multi-stake-holder arrangements in South India', *Cities* 24(2): 133–47

BrihanMumbai Municipal Corporation (2003) *Water Conservation & Rainwater Harvesting for BrihanMumbai*, Mumbai: BMC

Bulkeley, Harriet and Michele M. Betsill (2003) *Cities and Climate Change: Urban Sustainabiility and Global Environmental Governance*, London: Routledge

Bulkeley, Harriet and Heike Schroeder (2011) 'Beyond state/non-state divides: Global cities and the governing of climate change', *European Journal of International Relations* 18(4): 743–66

Button, Cat (2014) *Domesticating Infrastructure: Mumbai's Middle Class Housing and Rainwater Harvesting*, Department of Geography, Durham: Durham University

Button, Cat (2017) 'The co-production of a constant water supply in Mumbai's middle-class apartments', *Urban Research & Practice* 10(1): 102–19

Gandy, Matthew (2006) 'Water, Sanitation and the Modern City: Colonial and Post-colonial Experiences in Lagos and Mumbai'. Background paper written for the Human Development Report 2006, UNDP

Gandy, Matthew (2008) 'Landscapes of disaster: water, modernity, and urban fragmentation in Mumbai', *Environment and Planning A*, 40(1): 108–30

Graham, Stephen (2006) 'Urban metabolism as target: contempory war as forced demodernisation', in Nik Heynen, Maria Kaika and Erik Swyngedouw (eds.) *In the Nature of Cities: Urban Political Ecology and the Politics of Urban Metabolism*, London: Routledge, 245–65

Graham, Stephen, Renu Desai, and Colin McFarlane (2013) 'Water Wars in Mumbai', *Public Culture* 25(1): 115–41

Graham, Stephen and Simon Marvin (2001) *Splintering Urbanism: Networked Infrastructures, Technological Mobilities and the Urban Condition*, London: Routledge

Handia, Lubinga, James M. Tembo and Caroline Mwiindwa (2003) 'Potential of rainwater harvesting in urban Zambia', *Physics and Chemistry of the Earth, Parts A/B/C* 28(20–27): 893–6

Kahinda, Jean-marc, Akpofure E. Taigbenu and Jean R. Boroto (2007) 'Domestic rainwater harvesting to improve water supply in rural South Africa', *Physics and Chemistry of the Earth, Parts A/B/C* 32 (15–18): 1050–7

Kaika, Maria (2004) 'Interrogating the geographies of the familiar: domesticating nature and constructing the autonomy of the modern home', *International Journal of Urban and Regional Research* 28(2): 265–86

Kaika, Maria (2005) *City of Flows: Modernity, Nature, and the City*, London: Routledge

McFarlane, Colin (2008a) 'Sanitation in Mumbai's Informal Settlements: State, 'Slum', and Infrastructure', *Environment and Planning A* 40(1): 88–107

McFarlane, Colin (2008b) 'Urban shadows: materiality, the 'southern city' and urban theory', *Geography Compass* 2(2): 340–58

Municpal Corporation of Greater Mumbai (MCGM) (2008) 'Brihanmumbai Mahanagarpalika: Rain Water Harvesting', Mumbai: MCGM

Pandey, Deep N., Anil K. Gupta and David M. Anderson (2003) 'Rainwater harvesting as an adaptation to climate change', *CURRENT SCIENCE* 85(1): 46–59

Qayum, Seemin and Raka Ray (2011) 'The middle classes at home', in Amita Baviskar and Raka Ray (eds.) *Elite and Everyman: The cultural politics of the Indian middle class*, New Delhi: Routledge, 246–70

Shove, Elizabeth (2003) Comfort, *Cleanliness and Convenience: The Social Organization of Normality*, Oxford: Berg

Srivastava, Rahul and Matias Echanove (2014) '"Slum" is a loaded term. They are homegrown neighbourhoods', *The Guardian*, Friday 28 November

Sule, Surekha (no date) 'Mumbai's water supply', in N. Mukherjee (ed.) *Understanding our civic issues*, Mumbai: Bombay Community Public Trust

Swyngedouw, Erik (2004) *Social Power and the Urbanization of Water: Flows of Power*, Oxford: Oxford University Press

Trentmann, Frank (2009) 'Distribution is normal: blackouts, breakdowns and the elasticity of everyday life', in Elizabeth Shove, Frank Trentmann and Richard Wilk (eds.) *Time, Consumption and Everyday Life: Practice, Materiality and Culture*, Oxford: Berg, 67–84

Zérah, Marie-Hélène (2008) 'Splintering urbanism in Mumbai: contrasting trends in a multilayered society', *Geoforum* 39(6): 1922–32

CHAPTER 9

Transforming gender relations through water, sanitation, and hygiene programming and monitoring in Vietnam

Caitlin Leahy, Keren Winterford, Tuyen Nghiem,
John Kelleher, Lee Leong and Juliet Willetts

Abstract

This chapter presents the results of empirical research conducted in Central Vietnam in 2016 into water, sanitation, and hygiene (WASH) initiatives. It uncovered changes in gender relations and power dynamics at both household and community levels, aiming to explore the extent to which both practical and strategic interests of women can be influenced and changed by WASH policies and programming. In particular, we were interested in assessing the impact of a Gender and WASH Monitoring Tool (GWMT), developed by Plan International Australia and Plan Vietnam, on women's strategic gender needs. In this chapter, we discuss the types of changes reported by women and men of different ages and ethnicities and the reasons for their occurrence. There were a wide range of reported reasons for change, with implications for our understanding of the relationship between changes in gender relations at the household and community levels. We also consider the relationship between wider shifts in social norms in the context of rural Vietnam. The Vietnam research highlights the roles that WASH initiatives can play in furthering strategic gender needs and hence promoting gender equality and women's empowerment. It also shows the importance of addressing Sustainable Development Goal (SDG) 5 (on gender equality) and SDG 6 (on water and sanitation) together.

Keywords: Gender equality; gender outcomes; water; sanitation; hygiene; Vietnam

Introduction

This chapter aims to contribute to evidence of the ways in which water, sanitation, and hygiene (WASH) programmes can influence and change the underlying gender relations between men and women – and how the *strategic gender needs* of women can be met through a combination of WASH programming and effective monitoring. Strategic gender needs are defined as distinct from

http://dx.doi.org/10.3362/9781788530866.009

practical gender needs (based on the work on gender interests of Molyneux 1985), and a useful definition is provided by Moser (1993: 39, 40):

> Strategic gender needs are the needs women identify because of their subordinate position to men in their society. Strategic gender needs vary according to particular contexts. They relate to gender divisions of labour, power and control and may include such issues as legal rights, domestic violence, equal wages and women's control over their bodies. Meeting strategic gender needs helps women to achieve greater equality. It also changes existing roles and therefore challenges women's subordinate position.

> Practical gender needs are the needs women identify in their socially accepted roles in society. Practical gender needs do not challenge the gendered divisions of labour or women's subordinate position in society, although rising out of them. Practical gender needs are a response to immediate perceived necessity, identified within a specific context. They are practical in nature and often are concerned with inadequacies in living conditions such as water provision, health care, and employment.

This chapter draws on research in three locations in Central Vietnam to provide insights into how WASH programming implemented by district and commune-level government agencies, with the support of the international non-government organisation (NGO), Plan International[1] was able to contribute to meeting women's strategic gender needs.

WASH is not only a practical technical concern: lack of water and sanitation – and other basic needs – arises from complex societal inequalities, including gender inequality. At the level of policy, the relationship between poverty, deprivation, and inequalities is recognised in current global thinking on development. During the era of the Millennium Development Goals (MDGs) there was a growing awareness in the international community that to fulfil the ambition of safe water and sanitation for all, women's empowerment and gender equality needed to be addressed simultaneously (Willetts *et al.* 2010). The Sustainable Development Goals (SDGs) and the 2030 Agenda for Sustainable Development go further in many respects with a twin focus on basic needs and equal rights. However, this commitment still does not fully address issues of poverty and inequality together. While gender equality is the focus of the stand-alone 'gender goal', SDG 5, gender issues are also integrated to a varying extent into the other 16 goals. SDG 6, which aims to attain water and sanitation for all (implying women, men, girls, and boys), also explicitly mentions women and girls in Target 6.2, however, the relevant global indicators are not designed to capture gender differences adequately, since they focus on household, rather than intra-household, differences.

At the level of practice, gender mainstreaming efforts over the past two decades have attempted to integrate gender equality into sectors of development which focus on satisfying the practical needs of women and men living in poverty, including the need for water and sanitation. Many WASH programmes now also actively seek to make contributions to gender equality or women's empowerment outcomes, based on the realisation that WASH can be a strategic entry point for further change in gender relations (Carrard *et al.* 2013). Yet understanding of what this means, and in particular the need to focus on women's strategic needs, is not as widespread as it could be and the implications for programming are less well understood.

With this in mind, this chapter supports the idea that integration of SDGs 5 and 6 is essential, and offers insights here from our research in Vietnam to contribute to an evidence base on this. We hope that this will support WASH practitioners to develop their ability to work to address both practical and strategic gender needs, in an integrated way.

Research background: the empowering potential of WASH

From the early days of gender and development, it has been recognised that men and women will be affected differently by development initiatives, given their different socially constructed roles and responsibilities, opportunities, and constraints influenced by these, and the value placed on gendered roles and responsibilities. Women's interests relating to water and sanitation provision have a direct impact on the way they experience life, the tasks they perform, their potential, and the opportunities and difficulties they face (Fisher 2008). Women's practical needs (Moser 1989) can be met by furnishing women with resources, including water, sanitation, and hygiene, to meet needs arising from their positioning in the existing (unequal) gender division of labour. But in addition, women have a strategic gender interest (Molyneux 1985) in challenging gender inequality, which can be furthered by development interventions of various kinds.

The provision of safe clean water, sanitation, and hygiene affects women – and men – on both practical and strategic levels. Biological differences between women and men create gender-specific needs in relation to WASH. In addition to those health needs they share with men, women have a range of gender-specific health needs relating to reproductive and maternal health. These require WASH programming that includes menstrual hygiene management and the provision of safe water and sanitation facilities to improve outcomes for pregnant and new mothers and their babies (Tarrass and Benjelloun 2012).

In addition to these practical health needs, WASH also clearly has an impact on other practical needs of women arising from women's positioning in relation to men in society. Women typically perform care work for their households, ranging from water collection to preparing, cooking, and serving food and drinks, and delivering basic hygiene and health care to children and older people. Improving WASH conditions in households usually supports women in these unpaid domestic caregiving roles, linking to SDG 5's focus on caregiving and unpaid domestic work as a driver and a result of gender inequality (Razavi 2016).

In relation to violence against women and girls (VAWG), the distinction between practical and strategic needs is less clear. Women and girls are often at risk of violence when collecting water, bathing, or living in locations without adequate sanitation designed with safety in mind. Considerations such as facilities closer to home meet practical needs and can be very effective in reducing vulnerability to VAWG (House *et al.* 2014). Conversely, if WASH interventions are planned without considering such issues, they may result in programming that aggravates the problem of VAWG, rather than solving it, for example if women start to take on traditionally male roles in households or communities (*ibid*).

Above and beyond practical needs, WASH programmes can explicitly aim to address women's strategic gender needs. WASH has an impact at a strategic level in terms of the processes used in the planning and implementation of programming. WASH programming can further women's strategic gender interests, by supporting women's leadership and participation in development and governance (Willetts *et al.* 2010). Finally, WASH provisioning has potential to have a strategic impact on women and girls by freeing them to spend time in activities that bring material benefits, notably income generation or education, however, the global evidence base on these impacts is relatively weak and requires further research to prove with rigour.

Different authors writing specifically on WASH and empowerment vary in their view of the role of WASH programming in the empowerment of women. Saskia Ivens (2008) cautions against assuming that fulfilling practical needs of women leads to increased gender equality, pointing to a lack of evidence showing that advancement of women's access to water and participation in WASH-related decision-making has led to women's empowerment. In her work, Ivens draws on a United Nations Population Fund definition of empowerment, that it is identifying and redressing power imbalances in order to give women more autonomy to manage their own lives. Programming that delivers benefits for women may appear to be intrinsically empowering, but some studies show that if issues of power and the political nature of participation are not adequately considered in WASH-related decision-making bodies, women's influence will be limited (Kemerink *et al.* 2013).

Notwithstanding these cautionary comments, there is a growing recognition that WASH programming can provide an entry point for gender equality, and can lead to genuine shifts in power between women and men (Fisher 2008; Kilsby 2012; O'Reilly 2010; Willetts *et al.* 2010). To achieve these changes, however, requires a specific effort to use empowering and participatory approaches (Ivens 2008). Although she does not explicitly focus on WASH,[2] Naila Kabeer's (1999) model of empowerment conceptualises the provision of material resources to women as the starting point for a process whereby they are able to put their choices and aims into action, ultimately achieving empowerment.

It has been argued that within WASH programming, in particular, a comprehensive means of documenting and assessing strategic gender outcomes, as distinct from practical gender needs, has been lacking (Carrard *et al.* 2013). The case to address gender issues in WASH is often made on the grounds of enhanced efficiency instead of on the grounds of empowerment or gender equality as policy rationales. Since the 1970s and the UN Water Decade of the 1980s, there has been wide acknowledgement among development practitioners that when women and men are equally involved in WASH programmes, for example through equal and active participation in decisionmaking committees (commonly water management committees), the programmes can be made more effective and sustainable (Fisher 2008; Gross *et al.* 2000; O'Reilly 2010).

Despite a recognition that access to water and sanitation are human rights, there is a tendency in the WASH sector to target interventions to meet practical needs, with a focus on efficiency and sustainability of WASH outcomes, and the strategic needs that are linked to these are not often a central focus. However, there is growing realisation that these links need to be better understood, not least in light of the clearer link articulated in the SDG framework between gender equality and WASH.

The Gender and WASH Monitoring Tool

Against this backdrop, the GWMT was originally developed in 2011 by Plan International Australia and Plan Vietnam,[3] In 2011, discussions with other development agencies in Vietnam had highlighted that a number of agencies were facing similar challenges in monitoring strategic gender changes in communities where WASH programming was being implemented. It was proposed that a simple monitoring tool could help overcome this challenge. The GWMT duly aimed to monitor changes in gendered social norms, power relations, and the status of women and men (Thomas 2015). As Plan stated in its guide to the tool:

> Promoting gender equality demands significant attention in every WASH intervention as gender relations are integral to the effectiveness and sustainability of WASH. The literature suggests that measuring change in the context of gender relations presents ongoing challenges for monitoring and evaluation (M&E). (Plan International Australia 2014, 3)

The GWMT couples a regular monitoring activity with active exploration of gendered relations through a facilitated community dialogue process, to meet two aims. The first of these focuses on programme staff and partners, working at the community level on WASH and within government. The GWMT aims to support them to develop gender analysis skills and better understanding of the role that WASH can play in promoting gender equality. The second aim of the GWMT is to raise awareness among communities about gender roles and relationships in household and community WASH activities, and to promote aspirations for gender equality, providing opportunities for women and men to discuss gender relations, and to set their own agendas for change (*ibid.*).

Our research in Vietnam

Findings discussed in this paper draw on a 12-month study undertaken by the Institute for Sustainable Futures at the University of Technology, Sydney (ISF-UTS) in 2016 in collaboration with Plan International Australia, Plan Vietnam, and the Centre for Natural Resources and Environmental Studies (CRES) at the Vietnam National University. The research was designed to uncover women and men's perceptions of changes in gender relations in Central Vietnam, to determine whether the GWMT was directly contributing to the achievement of strategic gender outcomes. It aimed to explore the contribution of the GWMT (as well as WASH policies and programming) to changes in gender relations experienced during the duration of GWMT implementation.[4]

The research locations

Seven communities across three Central Provinces in Vietnam – Quảng Trị, Quảng Bình, and Kon Tum – were selected for inclusion in the research. These include ethnically diverse, remote mountainous regions. All villages were sites where Plan Vietnam had supported WASH interventions from 2012/13 until the time of the research and the focus of our research was to explore changes in gender relations over the period in which the GWMT had been implemented. Plan International Vietnam's WASH programming in these locations complements and supports the work of government. Partner institutions include district Centres for Preventative Medicine, the Departments of Agriculture and Rural Development, and local Women's Unions.

Programmes in these locations have included a number of components: community and school-based sanitation improvement and marketing of sanitation products[5]; school and community hygiene promotion and behaviour change communication; and water safety planning[6] and capacity-building to support community groups in operation and maintenance of WASH infrastructure. Gender and social inclusion components of the programme have included explicit gender equality objectives and targets, formative research on gender and inclusion, and a dedicated budget for gender-related activities. Separate WASH facilities are provided in schools for males and females, and menstrual hygiene management sessions are conducted in schools. Female representation in management and technical positions, trainees, and community meetings is between 30 and 52 per cent.

Research approach

The research used a conceptual framework – the Gender Outcomes Framework (GOF)[7] – which classifies gender equality changes associated with WASH programmes. The GOF aims to assist WASH practitioners and policymakers to more explicitly pursue strategic gender outcomes (that is, positive changes in gender power relations, in the direction of gender equality and women's empowerment) in WASH programming and policies. It aims to assist practitioners and researchers in designing programmes, monitoring, and documenting progress to achieve strategic gender outcomes (Carrard *et al.* 2013).

The GOF's design was used in the participatory processes employed for the research, and was also used to categorise, assess, and quantify the changes described by research participants. The GOF categorises the gender outcomes associated with WASH initiatives as relating either to individual changes or changes in relationships, and identifies three spheres within which these changes can occur. These are: the household sphere; the local public arena (that is, social and community networks); and the wider public arena (including governance institutions and beyond) (*ibid.*).

The research focused on a selected set of seven strategic gender outcomes that had been identified prior to the research (Figure 1). These were relevant to Plan's evaluation of the impact of its work in these areas of Central Vietnam. All affected gender relations in the household sphere or the local public arena. Changes in the wider public arena were not a focus for this research, since the GWMT is not directly aimed at this level. The research was carried out in awareness of the challenges of attribution in that change is complex and can never be wholly or directly linked to a single factor.

A range of social, economic, and environmental factors determine a person's experience of change. In recognition of this, the research disaggregated results by a number of these factors. These included gender, age, ethnicity, and location.

Research methods

In total, the research engaged 187 men and women: 48 participants in semi-structured interviews and 139 participants in pocket-voting. Participants in the research were selected by the Vietnamese research team from the

	Household sphere *Household and family networks*	Local public arena *Social and community networks*
Changes in self/individuals *Includes changes for women or men* *Includes changes relating to roles as well as self-perception and attitudes*	SGO1: Changes in the **distribution of household roles and labour** between women and men SGO2: Changes in **self-confidence**, particularly for women	SGO4: Changes in the number of women occupying public and potentially influential **roles** in their community SGO5: Changes in **self-confidence**, including to participate in community meetings/forums, particularly for women
Changes in relationships *Includes changes in relationships between women/men and within gender groups*	SGO3: Changes in **communication** between household members in relation to influencing decision-making	SGO6: Changes in **solidarity** within and between women and men as collective groups SGO7: Changes in the extent to which women's perspectives are **listened to** at the community level

Figure 1. The strategic gender outcomes (SGOs) selected for exploration in this research.

CRES researchers who applied random sampling to GWMT participant lists obtained from Plan Vietnam and population lists obtained from government. Participants comprised 92 men and 95 women; people of different ethnic groups (Vân Kiều, Mó Nâm, and Kinh), younger people aged 18–30 and adults aged over 30, and three people living with disabilities participated in the research.

Semi-structured interviews used open-ended questions to encourage people to share particular experiences of gender-related change in relation to management of WASH activities in their households and communities during the time period that the GWMT had been implemented. Interviews were conducted by CRES researchers with individual men and women in a private setting and lasted approximately one hour. Probing questions helped to uncover the strategic outcomes people had experienced. Researchers then asked participants directly about the reasons that they thought such changes had occurred. For those participants who had taken part in the GWMT, a final question asked them to rate the level of influence the GWMT had on the gender-related changes they had experienced. Responses derived from these interviews formed the basis of detailed analysis which was complemented by the results of a pocket voting process.

A quantitative 'pocket voting' method invited groups of men and women to cast votes individually and in secret based on their experiences and perceptions of changes in relation to six of the seven strategic gender outcomes in the home and community. They voted that they had experienced 'a lot of change', 'no change', or 'a little change'. These categories cannot reveal the extent of change that was needed: context-specific and detailed analysis is needed beyond this relatively simple tool to give an indication of progress. For this reason, pocket voting results served as a rough gauge of progress to complement the detailed analysis of responses derived through the semi-structured interviews. Voting results were revealed and participants were asked direct questions based on results. They were invited to report on their own first-hand experience or their observations of change happening around them. The discussions with groups of women and groups of men also revealed people's thinking about the reasons for change taking place or not over the period of GWMT implementation. A wider discussion with both women and men together then provided a space to compare analyses, share experiences and perceptions, and discuss possible explanations for these. Analysis of the findings was conducted using quantitative and qualitative tools,[8] and the research was approved through the ISF-UTS university ethics approval process.[9]

Research findings

Selected findings of the research are presented here in order to paint a picture of the gender change uncovered in the research sites, the different experiences of groups within the research, and the reasons given for why change happened. Complete findings of the research, including in relation to the impact of the GWMT can be found in Caitlin Leahy *et al.* (2016).

In relation to amount of change, the research revealed participants' perceptions that considerable change had occurred in gender relations. Most of this was positive – that is, gender relations were now more equal and women more empowered – although there were some examples of negative change taking place. Thirty-nine of the 48 participants interviewed (that is, 81 per cent) described at least one change over the previous three years that indicated a positive shift in power relations between men and women. In addition, pocket voting results revealed that these results were widespread, and not confined to the interview sample frame. On average, 68 per cent of all votes cast by both women (72) and men (67) were cast for 'a lot of change' in relation to each of the six strategic gender outcomes identified at household and community levels.

Experiences of different gender, age, and ethnic groups

Over three-quarters of research participants, of both sexes (78 per cent of women and 84 per cent of men) reported during interviews that they had experienced at least one of the six strategic gender outcomes identified for the research. However, pocket voting discussions revealed qualitative data showing gendered differences in perceptions of change, and assessments of how empowered women were (or had become). For example, in three villages, discussion revealed that women perceived themselves to have become either more or less self-confident than men perceived them to be. This highlights the importance of hearing from both women and men separately in any efforts to understand gender changes.

Participants in the 18–30 age group reported more change than the older (30+) age group (91 per cent compared with 72 per cent). One possible explanation for this is that young people may be experiencing change for the first time and therefore talk openly about their experience. Younger people also sometimes described change in relation to their parents or grandparents as a point of difference. In regards to ethnicity, compared to the Kinh majority, participants in the Mó Nâm and Vân Kiêu ethnic groups more commonly reported strategic gender outcomes (56 per cent Kinh, 95 per cent Vân Kiêu, and 92 per cent Mó Nâm). This was despite the fact that particular customary or cultural norms were reported by Vân Kiêu women and men as barriers to change in the division of labour, particularly at the household level. One younger Vân Kiêu man describes this as follows:

> Our Vân Kiêu ethnic people are used to distributing all housework to their wives, men have never washed clothes because they are shy, and they are afraid that someone else would see them wash clothes. (Interview, Tà Lêng village, 9 May 2016)

Examples of positive and negative change reported

The research revealed that experiences of change were more commonly reported at the household level, rather than the community level, a finding demonstrated through both interview responses (59 per cent of outcomes were reported at the household level compared with 40 per cent reported at the community level) and pocket voting results (55 per cent of all votes for 'change a lot' were for household-level changes compared with 45 per cent at the community level).

The most commonly reported outcome experienced at the household level was improved communication between male and female household members, in which women increased their influence over decision-making. A total of 39 per cent of women and 48 per cent of men reported such a change. The following example was described by one younger Kinh man:

> Before, making decision who work what in the family belonged to me, my wife do all houseworking, and cut grass near the house, husband go to the forest, field. Now, I and my wife discuss all works, sometime she makes the decision. (Interview, Tà Lêng village, 9 May 2016)

The next most commonly reported outcome experienced at the household level was women's increased self-confidence in intra-household relations. A change of this nature was reported by 35 per cent of women and 28 per cent of men, including this example given by one younger Vân Kiều woman:

> Compared with three or four years ago, I changed a lot, I am self-confident to talk out what I want or don't want. I dare to ask my husband to sweep house or wash up, take a bath for babies whenever I am busy, and my husband is happy to do that. (Interview, Ly Tôn village, 11 May 2016)

At the community level, the most common outcome reported was a change in women's self-confidence, including self-confidence to participate in community meetings or forums. Overall, 35 per cent of women and 44 per cent of men interviewed for the research reported examples of this type of change. One younger Vân Kiều woman reported that:

> Women have more self-confidence. They speak up more often. They were reluctant to speak up before because they were afraid of men criticizing. Women can say that men are wrong and ask for help. Recently they asked men in the village to fix water pipes because they are too tired to do it. They used to be too shy to talk to men. But now they meet and talk to men many times they are not shy anymore. (Interview, Ly Tôn village, 11 May 2016)

In relation to women's occupation of public and influential roles, many examples were given of women attending meetings, with a small number of examples given of women in leadership roles. During interviews, 26 per cent of women and 28 per cent of men reported such changes. Some examples referred to women increasingly taking part in 'communal works' such as village cleaning or construction, cleaning, and maintenance of public water sources. These examples tended to suggest a more shared public work role between men and women – suggesting a positive change in gender relations that empowers women – rather than women simply taking on the burden of communal work. As reported by one older Kinh woman:

> Before, the leader of clusters were mostly men, now, many cluster leaders are women. They mobilise the masses to clean up the village road and invite the men to participate. They give their ideas more. (Interview, Cây Dâu village, 6 May 2016)

Some negative changes were reported by participants. A total of 101 changes in gender relations were reported during interviews, of which eight changes were negative. All but one of the participants reporting negative changes also reported positive changes during their interviews. This reminds us that change to gender relations is not a linear, simple process. Three younger Vân Kiều women reported negative changes involving an increase in men's drinking. One explanation for this was an increase in standards of living, which resulted in men drinking and not wanting to help with other activities.

One of these women stated that:

> … before, the men in this village sometimes also helped their wife to do houseworking, [but] some years recently, they do nothing, they are so lazy, they only drink all the time with each other, they don't hear any advice. (Interview, Khe Ngài village, 13 May 2016)

What factors contributed to positive change in gender relations?

Social change is complex, and attributing it to particular factors can be subjective. Participants involved in the research gave accounts which included their own opinions on the reasons for change. Of all changes which emerged in the research, nearly one-third (31 per cent) appeared, through our analysis, to be directly attributable to a WASH process, policy, or outcome. The remainder were linked to a broader set of factors and participants provided a range of interlinking reasons for why change had taken place in households and communities. This example, provided by an older Kinh woman, illustrates her perception of the role of targeted WASH interventions as these are situated among broader societal factors:

> The women now are more self-confident, they are so active in ordering people to participate in cleaning up [the] village road, to keep it more clean. They dare to give more ideas at the meetings, when the men give ideas that they don't feel comfortable with, they will ask again. Before, whenever the women's association had meetings, there were many women did not participate or they gave up the meeting when the

meeting was not finished, because of the low education and poverty. [Change happened] because of the lifestyle, before, the women were not treated well, the life was so poor, they were hard working, now the living standard is better, the women are trained more, have more knowledge. Three or four years ago, when Plan introduced the community to do WASH, they integrated to introduce the women to know about the women's right, every house see each other to live better, every one more pay attention. (Interview, Hát village, 3 May 2016)

The contribution of WASH to change in gender relations

The specific WASH interventions cited by participants as contributing to positive change in gender relations are outlined here in order, from most reported to least reported.

In the three contexts we studied, WASH programming was found to have equipped women with information and knowledge, particularly technical knowledge, which contributed to them having a voice in decision-making in homes and communities. This strategy was shown in all three settings to be effective in relation to WASH-specific information and more general access to education and training. WASH-specific activities feed into wider processes of public information and peer-to-peer learning that are occurring in the broader context.

The most reported example of this was WASH meetings and training – either technical WASH-related training (how to build and maintain a toilet, a water tank, or water pipes; the benefit of using soap in hand washing; clean water) or specific training offered to both women and men on gender equality and rights.

Whilst the space given for women to share ideas and gain confidence was seen as important, access to technical information in itself was also a key factor because this allowed women to more confidently negotiate about roles and decisions in the home. One older Vân Kiều woman explained:

> My husband used to decide everything in our home. But he listened to me and built the toilet because I told him that it made it easy for all of us when it rains, and that I could tell him how to build a toilet. (Interview, Tà Lêng village, 9 May 2016)

An improvement in WASH-related infrastructure at the household or community level (e.g. new water pipes, a communal water tank, or a new toilet) was also identified as an important contributing factor that had brought about positive changes in gender relations within marriage and the family. An improvement in WASH infrastructure had, for example, changed the nature of household work, leading to a reduction in the workload associated with domestic water use, and sometimes encouraging men to take on some of this work – thereby redistributing roles in the household more equally between women and men.

However, it is also important to note that an improvement in WASH infrastructure does not necessarily change power dynamics between women and men. It may even increase women's workload in particular contexts, underlining the importance of careful research at the programme-planning stage to ensure this does not happen. An older Kinh man described the increased workload of his wife after they gained access to a water well:

> The difference is in the past everyone bathed at the stream and did their own clothes washing. Now when we have a water well, my wife do laundry for everyone. My wife does laundry for all at the same time for saving detergent. (Interview, Hát village, 4 May 2016)

The involvement of leaders and figures of authority in WASH programmes or strategies was also identified as contributing to changes. These people can encourage equal participation of women and men in WASH activities (including meetings), and can help raise awareness of the importance of gender equality in households and communities. Although a change brought about by an authoritative command may not signal a genuine shift in gender relations, the research identified that where this brought about initial participation by women in community meetings or activities, it could lead to more sustained participation as a result of the growing confidence of women.

For example, one younger Mó Nâm man observed that:

> [The] reason for more participation of woman is: a woman goes to a meeting, the woman gets to know others, so she is more self-confident. The more participation, the more happy the women are because they can talk more about works and business. (Interview, Kon Leng 2 village, 18 May 2016)

Interestingly, the research did not find a direct link between the use of the GWMT and the achievement of strategic gender outcomes. However, use of the GWMT could be seen as a way to reinforce and bring visibility to efforts made in WASH programming to support gender equality.

The contribution of other factors to gendered change

Importantly, nearly two-thirds (69 per cent) of reasons for strategic gender outcomes described by participants were mainly attributable to a wide range of other factors. This is not a surprising result and suggests that WASH interventions need to be seen in the context of broad, ongoing social, economic, and political factors that will influence social relations, including gender relations. It also reinforces the importance of research methodology that is not based on a skewed understanding of the role of planned development in contributing to broader change. Development practitioners and policymakers need to genuinely understand this if they are to ensure their planned interventions, in WASH and in other sectors, are to contribute to the continuous broader trends of challenge and change to gender relations.

The range of factors that came up in the research as responsible for positive change in gender relations is briefly outlined here in order, from most reported to least reported. Some factors echoed similar WASH-specific factors.

The most common factor was increased access to information and education, particularly for women. Both formal and non-formal channels were identified, including formal schooling and training but also public information – referred to by some as 'propaganda', as in the example that follows below. This information was conveyed in various channels including through public announcements and television, and peer-to-peer learning. The impact was described as both enabling women to become more knowledgeable and also increasing women's and men's (and boys' and girls') understanding about gender equality. One younger Mó Nâm woman shared her experience that:

> I found my husband often help me more in housework. Thanks to propaganda, my husband and son understand that they have to help me. (Interview, Kon Leng 2 village, 18 May 2016)

Such public education is provided by Vietnam Women's Union and local officials. Several participants (mostly from the two ethnic minorities) referred to 'cadre' which can mean government figures but can also mean other important figures outside government).

Another younger Vân Kiều woman reported the influence of other women, in particular older women, in development terminology; this would be seen as 'peer-to-peer learning':

> I am more self-confident because I learnt from my mother and others. I found they can do it [ask for husband's help], so I also do it. (Interview, Khe Ngài village, 13 May 2016)

This example is interesting in that it goes against the notion that change happens when people challenge ideas that have been passed on by parents and older people to accept, thereby associating younger people with change. In fact, individuals may be influenced by many factors to challenge gendered social norms and beliefs, and change can therefore flow in different ways between the generations.

Individual attitudes and values were also identified as contributing to change. This may have referred to personal convictions (to act against customs and norms), a desire to avoid conflict, empathy, and love, leading to a change in power dynamics between women and men. This is demonstrated by this older Vân Kiều man's example:

> Now I help my wife more than before. My wife does a lot of work (weeding, sweeping the house, cooking ...) so I wash clothes. Everybody here says that I'm afraid of my wife but I don't care. I help her because I love her. (Interview, Ly Tôn village, 11 May 2016)

Sometimes a necessity or practicality effected a change in household roles, and had a positive impact on gender equality in the process. One younger Vân Kiều women reported her increased self-confidence as a result of a change in household composition:

> Four years ago, since I moved to live independently, I was more forcible and less shy because we had common children and my husband must help to take care of the children. (Interview, Khe Ngài village, 13 May 2016)

Over and above these reasons cited for change, the impact of broader changes in society on gender equality outcomes came out strongly in the responses provided by participants. Examples referred to a range of factors: generational change; influences from outside the village; increased living standards; television and media; and the influence of social norms in wider society. This broader set of factors was reported as leading to changes in roles and decision-making in households, changes in self-confidence of women in the community, and the number of women in public roles. One older Kinh man described the impact of wider social norms on roles of women and men in the household and community:

> Many men go to work outside. They found men and women are equal there, and applied at home. (Interview, Hát village, 4 May 2016)

Another man also suggested that:

> Women in this village often strongly remind their husbands to help them with housework. Because it is the right thing to do. They learn that from society. (Pocket voting discussion, Cây Dâu village, 6 May 2016)

How can greater gender change be achieved through WASH interventions?

This research confirms that WASH interventions have a significant role to play in supporting gender equality and women's empowerment in Central Vietnam. Here, and further afield, WASH practitioners can learn from what has worked in a particular context, and thereby seek to increase their impact.

As stated earlier, there is an evidence gap in the documentation of the impact of WASH programmes on gender relations, at the level of strategic gender outcomes. However, findings from this research are broadly consistent with a later study in Timor-Leste which drew on the same methodology and identified a range of factors bringing about strategic gender change (Kilsby 2012). Factors that were similar to those found in our study included: 'information', understood to include information about water and sanitation options, and possibly about women's rights to participate; women's participation in meetings, which enabled change to take place both in terms of substantive issues considered and perceptions about the value of women's participation;

a recognition within the community that allowing women greater rights is the right thing to do; access to new facilities (clean water closer to home and sanitation facilities) led to men doing more of the work (Kilsby 2012). Other factors found in the Timor-Leste study (Kilsby 2012) which were less commonly reported in our research included: women in new roles acting as role models for others; funds and technical support from NGOs; and women staff working in communities.

Strategies to address gender equality need to consider using specific approaches relevant for people of different ages and ethnicities. Identifying generational, cultural, and customary barriers to achieving gender equality outcomes and recognising the nuances in these is an important step. Participants described the process of adopting behaviours or values they saw taking shape in wider society into their local context, and this may be built upon through WASH programming in contexts where strong generational, cultural, and customary barriers exist.

Recognising the particular role that men play in bringing about positive change in gender relations is crucial for WASH practitioners. The most commonly reported of the four strategic gender outcomes focusing on life in the community was women's increased selfconfidence. In contrast, the least commonly reported of the four strategic gender outcomes was 'changes in solidarity within and between women and men' and 'changes in the extent to which women's perspectives are listened to at the community level'. This shows that changes are needed in men's perceptions of women, and in particular their views on the worth of women's community-level participation. Hence, WASH programmes need to work with boys and men in ways that consider their particular gendered relationships with women in households and communities, and ensure they are as supportive as possible to the aims of gender equality and the empowerment of women. Given that our research also found that men and women's perceptions of change differed, it is particularly important to give space within programmes for men and women to discuss their different aspirations and experiences separately, and subsequently together, in a facilitated process such as the GWMT.

As stated above, the research also revealed some negative changes in gender relations. Some were related to WASH programming, as in the example of the woman who was now washing clothes for her whole household. Other examples were less clearly attributable to WASH programming. This highlights that practitioners need to be aware not only of the complex and non-linear nature of change, but also the importance of mitigating unintended negative impacts on gender equality outcomes as a result of, for example, improving access to WASH infrastructure. Holding community meetings and discussions which take power imbalances into account can help to ensure that women do not shoulder the burden of additional workloads.

While the research did not find a direct link between the current use of the GWMT and the achievement of strategic gender outcomes, we think the use of such a monitoring tool may reinforce and support changes prompted by

WASH programming. Monitoring tools which make a clear distinction between practical changes and strategic changes have greater potential to inform an approach to programming which addresses unequal gender relations. The GWMT also ensures WASH programmes are prompted to include processes that this research has shown to be valid and important. These include making specific efforts to include women in discussions; separating women and men for relevant activities by age (to recognise the different experiences of younger and older people); targeting some households who can then set examples that have a positive flow-on effect; and helping people explore their perceptions and expectations of change. Furthermore, gender-responsive monitoring tools can be used as an important capacity-building approach for programme staff and partners.

Conclusion

The empirical research from Vietnam outlined in this paper reinforces the observation that WASH interventions can and do successfully contribute to gender equality outcomes – at both the practical and strategic level and in both the household and local community spheres. Recognition that WASH programming is an entry point to achieving gender equality is critical for delivering both SDG 5 on gender equality and SDG 6 on water and sanitation. However, this depends on the explicit use of contextually appropriate strategies to bring about genuine changes in power dynamics and increased gender equality through programming and monitoring. Making the distinction between practical and strategic gender needs in the design, implementation, and monitoring of WASH programmes, including through the use of the GWMT, provides a significant opportunity to ensure that WASH programmes are going beyond an approach that includes women on the grounds of efficiency, or claim aims of gender equality without a real understanding of how to achieve this. If WASH practitioners only focus on meeting the practical needs of women – as important as they may be – or see the inclusion of women (without any attention to assessing the rationale, the quality, or the outcomes of that inclusion) as 'good practice' for sustainable interventions, they will fall short of what they can potentially do on gender equality and the empowerment of women. Seeing WASH programming as an entry point to achieve gender equality provides an important opportunity to integrate SDG 5 and SDG 6 effectively.

Notes

1. For further information on Plan International, see: www.plan.org.au/learn/how-we-work/resources.
2. Much of the literature on empowerment of women that emerged in the mid-1990s onwards actually focused on micro-finance, a sector recognised more widely than WASH as a sector where immediate material

and economic need was addressed via activities that could potentially challenge gender power relations and social norms. Much literature on the empowerment potential of development programming focused on the potential of micro-finance to move beyond its immediate economic goals to support women's empowerment and gender equality (Kabeer 1998).

3. For full information, see www.plan.org.au/~/media/plan/documents/resources/gwmt-march-2014.pdf (last checked 16 March 2017).

4. The study was funded by the Australian Government, Department of Foreign Affairs and Trade, under the Innovation and Impact Fund of the Civil Society Water, Sanitation and Hygiene Fund (CS WASH Fund).

5. Sanitation marketing refers to the development of enterprises who utilise a marketing approach to sell sanitation products and services, with the aim of increasing latrine coverage in communities and/or institutions.

6. Water safety planning refers to interventions which reduce the risks of contamination to water sources from point source to use/disposal.

7. The framework draws on research carried out by ISF-UTS and the International Women's Development Agency in 2009–2011 (Halcrow et al. 2010). It was developed by Naomi Carrard and Juliet Willetts from ISF-UTS. For more information, see Carrard et al. (2013).

8. A quantitative approach was used to 'count' the gender outcomes reported by participants to see differences in the experiences of strategic gender outcomes across the different groups. ISF-UTS presented initial quantitative analysis during the collaborative data analysis workshop with partners in order to validate findings and gain contextual insights and explanations. A qualitative analysis of interview transcripts was also undertaken. Within the scope of the strategic outcomes framework, a thematic analysis was used to define how the strategic gender outcomes were experienced in the context of rural Vietnam and the influencing factors for this change.

9. Ethical design was informed by the ACFID 'Principles and Guidelines for Ethical Research and Evaluation in Development', including respect for human beings, research merit and integrity, beneficence, and justice (ACFID 2016). Partners involved in data collection on the ground were trained in these principles and processes.

Notes on contributors

Caitlin Leahy is a Senior Research Consultant at the Institute for Sustainable Futures at the University of Technology, Sydney (ISF-UTS). Email: Caitlin.Leahy@uts.edu.au

Keren Winterford is a Research Director at the Institute for Sustainable Futures at the University of Technology, Sydney (ISF-UTS). Email: Keren.Winterford@uts.edu.au

Tuyen Nghiem is a Senior Researcher at the Centre for Natural Resources and Environmental Studies at the Vietnam National University. Email: tuyennghiem_cres@yahoo.com

John Kelleher is Senior Program Manager WASH at Plan International Australia. Email: John.Kelleher@plan.org.au

Lee Leong Senior Advisor WASH at Plan International Australia. Email: Lee.Leong@plan.org.au

Juliet Willetts is a Professor and Research Director at the Institute for Sustainable Futures at theUniversity of Technology, Sydney (ISF-UTS). Email: Juliet.Willetts@uts.edu.au

References

ACFID (2016) *Principles and Guidelines for ethical research and evaluation in development*, Deakin, ACT: Australian Council for International Development, https://acfid.asn.au/sites/site.acfid/files/resource_document/Principles-for-Ethical-Research-and-Evaluation-in-Development2016.pdf (last checked 6 June 2017)

Carrard, Naomi, Joanne Crawford, Gabrielle Halcrow, Claire Rowland and Juliet Willetts (2013) 'A framework for exploring gender equality outcomes from WASH programmes', *Waterlines: International Journal of Water, Sanitation and Waste* 32(4): 315–333

Fisher, Julie (2008) 'Women in water supply, sanitation and hygiene programmes', *Proceedings of the ICE: Municipal Engineer* 161(4): 223–229

Gross, Bruce, Christine van Wijk and Nilanjana Mukherjee (2000) *Linking Sustainability with Demand, Gender and Poverty: A Study in Ccommunity-managed Water Supply Projects in 15 Countries*, Delft: Water and Sanitation Program, https://www.wsp.org/sites/wsp.org/files/publications/global_plareport.pdf (last checked 6 June 2017)

Halcrow, Gabrielle, Claire Rowland, Juliet Willetts, Joanne Crawford and Naomi Carrard (2010) *Resource Guide: Working effectively with women and men in water, sanitation and hygiene programs*, Melbourne: IWDA and ISF-UTS

House, Sarah, Suzanne Ferron, Marni Sommer and Sue Cavill (2014) *Violence, Gender & WASH: A Practitioner's Toolkit – Making Water, Sanitation and Hygiene Safer through Improved Programming and Services*, London, UK: WaterAid/SHARE

Ivens, Saskia (2008) 'Does increased water access empower women?' Development 51: 63–67

Kabeer, Naila (1998) 'Jumping to conclusions: struggles over meaning and method in the study of household economics', in Cecile Jackson and Ruth Pearson (eds.) *Feminist Visions of Development: Gender Analysis and Policy*, London: Routledge, 91–107

Kabeer, Naila (1999) *The Conditions and Consequences of Choice: Reflections on the Measurement of Women's Empowerment.* UNRISD Discussion Paper No. 108, August, Geneva: United Nations Research Institute for Social Development

Kemerink, Jeltsje Sanne, Linda Esteli Méndez, Rhodante Ahlers, Phillipus Wester and Pieter van der Zaag (2013) 'The question of inclusion and representation in rural South Africa: challenging the concept of water user associations as a vehicle for transformation', *Water Policy* 15(2): 243–57

Kilsby, Di (2012) *Now we feel like respected adults: Positive change in gender roles and relations in a Timor-Leste WASH programme*, ACFID Research in

Development Series, Report No. 6, Deakin, ACT: International Women's Development Agency, WaterAid, and Australian Council for International Development

Leahy, C., K. Winterford, J. Kelleher, L. Leong, T. Nghiem, N.Q. Hoa, and J. Willetts (2016) 'From practical to strategic changes: Strengthening gender in WASH.' *Final research report, prepared by Institute for Sustainable Futures*, University of Technology Sydney

Molyneux, Maxine (1985) 'Mobilization without Emancipation? Women's Interests, the State and Revolution in Nicaragua', *Feminist Studies* 11(2): 227–54

Moser, Caroline (1989) 'Gender planning in the third world: Meeting practical and strategic gender needs', *World Development* 17(11): 1799–1825

Moser, Caroline (1993) *Gender Planning and Development: Theory, Practice and Training*, London and New York: Routledge

O'Reilly, Kathleen (2010) 'Combining sanitation and women's participation in water supply: an example from Rajasthan', *Development in Practice* 20(1): 45–56

Plan International Australia (2014) 'Gender and WASH Monitoring Tool', Southbank, VIC: Plan International Australia, https://www.plan.org.au/~/media/plan/documents/resources/gwmt-march-2014.pdf (last checked 6 June 2017)

Razavi, Shahra (2016) 'The 2030 Agenda: challenges of implementation to attain gender equality and women's rights', *Gender & Development* 24(1): 25–41

Tarrass, Faissal and Meryem Benjelloun (2012) 'The effects of water shortages on health and human development', *Perspectives in Public Health* 132(5): 240–4

Thomas, E. (2015) 'Review of the Gender WASH Monitoring Tool (GWMT), Final Report', Plan Vietnam and Plan Australia

Willetts, Juliet, Gabrielle Halcrow, Naomi Carrard, Claire Rowland and Jo Crawford (2010) 'Addressing two critical MDGs together: gender in water, sanitation and hygiene initiatives', *Pacific Economic Bulletin* 25(1): 162–176

CHAPTER 10

'Breaking the silence around menstruation': experiences of adolescent girls in an urban setting in India

Shobhita Rajagopal and Kanchan Mathur

Abstract

The onset of menstruation is one of the important changes that occur in the lives of adolescent girls. It brings many challenges with it. Menstruation is often dealt with in secrecy in many cultures and communities. In India, restrictions are placed on women and girls during menstruation, and the tradition of excluding menstruating women and girls from various activities continues. Adolescent girls also suffer from myriad health problems associated with menstruation. Many lack the facilities and resources they need for menstrual hygiene. This chapter draws on research into the experiences and challenges faced by adolescent girls in managing menstruation at school and home in the slums of Jaipur, Rajasthan. The chapter analyses the role and impact of government-led policy and interventions. It argues that the continued silence around menstruation needs to be broken: not only by addressing the practical issues of menstrual management, but also by creating a supportive environment for empowering girls with information about their bodies, and destigmatising the issue of menstruation. The chapter also draws lessons for policy advocacy.

Keywords: Menstruation; menstrual hygiene; silence; adolescent girls; taboos; empowerment

Introduction

> When I started menstruating I was not prepared for it. No one had talked to me about menstrual blood, at home or in school. When I told my mother that I had blood stains on my underwear, I was advised to use cloth, and not enter the temple or touch pickle. I usually miss a day or two of school during my period. (Rita, 15 years old, focus group discussion with schoolgirls in Jaipur city, June 2016)

The onset of menstruation, and the practices associated with it, are areas shrouded in silence across many cultures in South Asia; yet they bring many

http://dx.doi.org/10.3362/9781788530866.010

challenges. On the one hand, puberty is a period of rapid transition for adolescent girls, and a critical time for identity formation; on the other, prevailing patriarchal ideologies, cultural taboos, and traditional practices exclude women and girls from various activities, including school attendance, reinforcing gender inequalities.

A number of recent studies have focused on knowledge, attitude, and practices regarding menstruation and hygiene in India (including Dube and Sharma 2012; Khanna *et al*. 2005; Sahayog 2016). They confirm a widespread silence around girls' experience of menstruation and puberty, and highlight that the impact of this on girls themselves is far-ranging. Attitudes too are generally unsupportive, and girls grow up in environments where there are a range of practical challenges including unmet water, sanitation, and hygiene (WASH) and health needs. Managing the practical and psychological aspects of menstruation is difficult for girls, affecting self-confidence and self-esteem, and the achievement of the wider development goal of women's empowerment. In particular, unmet menstrual hygiene needs affect girls' sense of 'power within', and their 'power to' – placing constraints on their mobility and the activities they can do – in particular, education.

Studies emphasise a need to focus on menstruation, challenging the stigma that surrounds it, and focusing also on practical aspects of how to manage menstruation – referred to in the literature most often as 'menstrual hygiene'.[1] Recent policy directives issued by the Government of India (2015) emphasise the need to raise awareness around menstrual hygiene management to empower adolescent girls.

> Good menstrual hygiene is crucial for the health, education, and dignity of girls and women. Equipping adolescent girls with adequate information and skills on menstrual hygiene and its management helps in empowering them with knowledge which enhances their self-esteem and positively impacts academic performance. It is important that the wider society, communities and families must challenge the status quo and break the silence around menstruation. (Government of India 2015, 5)

Menstrual health and hygiene is part of the National Health Mission, the flagship programme of the Government of India launched in 2005. The primary focus has been on raising awareness on menstrual hygiene. Distribution of subsidised disposable sanitary napkins[2] for adolescent girls in the rural areas is also part of the programme (Ministry of Health and Family Welfare, Government of India 2016).

This chapter draws on a study of a recent scheme, UDAAN ('We Fly'), launched in July 2015 for rural areas of Rajasthan but also covering poor urban areas of Jaipur. While assessing the impact of UDAAN, the study focused more widely on the experiences and continued challenges faced by adolescent girls in managing menstruation, and the need to break the silence around menstruation.

Setting the context: gender, education, and health in Rajasthan

Rajasthan is one of the largest states in northern India. It ranks eighth in terms of total population among Indian states (Government of Rajasthan 2016, 1) and has a large rural population. Jaipur, its capital, has an estimated 3.5 million inhabitants, of whom 22.4 per cent live in the city's slums (PFI 2012).

Gender-based inequalities in Rajasthan are acute. Gender differentials in literacy are also high: male literacy is 79.19 per cent, while female literacy is just 52.12 per cent (Government of Rajasthan 2016, 98). The average age of completion for elementary school for boys and girls is 14 years. While elementary education (Grades 1–8) statistics are improving and the gender gap is narrowing, the drop-out rate of girls is higher compared to boys (U-DISE 2014–15 2015). In addition, despite improvements at elementary levels, gender disparity at higher levels of schooling is a persisting development challenge, with serious consequences for empowerment of girls. The overall percentage of girls in total enrolment in secondary education in Rajasthan is 41.60 per cent; at the secondary stage it is 42.60 per cent and at the higher secondary stage it is 40.66 per cent (Rajagopal and Sharma 2016, 9). The gender gap at secondary level is 12.56 per cent (U-DISE 2016–17 raw data provided by Rajasthan Council of Secondary Education, Government of Rajasthan).

Schooling through adolescence and beyond offers girls an option beyond early marriage and childbearing. Rajasthan has a high prevalence of child marriage. The percentage of girls who are married before the legal age of 18 years is 31.6 per cent, as compared to the national figure of 17 per cent (Government of Rajasthan 2017, 4). This means that a high percentage of adolescent girls enter motherhood at an early age; with far-reaching health implications.

While the overall health indicators for Rajasthan have shown some improvement in the past decade, many challenges continue, and these include challenges relating to maternal and child health. The maternal mortality rate for the state was 244, much higher than the India national average of 167 (NitiAyog 2017). The recent National Family Health Survey (2015–16, 2) indicates that the fertility rate declined from 3.2 in 2005–06 to 2.4 in 2015–16. However, it continues to be higher than the average for India of 2.2 (*ibid.*, 2). The report also states that nearly half – 46.8 per cent – of women in the 15–49 years age group are anaemic (*ibid.*, 4); and that Infant Mortality Rate fell from 65 in 2007 to 41 in 2015–16, but this is still high compared to other Indian states (*ibid.*, 2).

Adolescent girls's experience of menstruation in Rajasthan

Barriers to adolescent girls' education include unmet WASH needs, including those related to menstruation. Various studies carried out in Rajasthan (Dube and Sharma 2012; Khanna *et al.* 2005) have assessed adolescent girls' knowledge and attitudes about reproductive health and menstrual practices. They note a huge knowledge gap among adolescent girls regarding menstrual processes. Years of schooling, residential status, caste, and exposure to media are major factors in adolescent girls and women's adoption of safe and hygienic menstrual practices (*ibid.*). The issues are worst in the rural areas, where a few non-government organisations (NGOs) (e.g. Jatan Sansthan and Vishakha) have initiated safe menstrual health campaigns and body awareness programmes in schools and local communities. They have also produced a range of washable and reusable sanitary napkins.[3]

Fear and panic is a dominant reaction reported by many girls in these studies at the time of their first periods. Much of the information imparted to a young girl about puberty and menstruation focuses on the need to restrict her movements and modify her behaviour. Female mobility is widely constrained due to social and cultural norms, but lack of reliable, efficient, and discreet means of dealing with menstruation present an additional practical set of issues. Girls frequently missed school for one or two days during their menstrual period. The silence around the issue within homes also transmits into educational institutions; this is not a topic dealt with openly in schools. The majority of the girls in the rural areas focused on in the studies used old cloths as protection, and many reported suffering from various reproductive health problems (Dube and Sharma 2012; Khanna *et al.* 2005).[4]

Similar issues exist in Rajasthan's urban areas. Maya Unnithan-Kumar conducted an ethnographic study (Unnithan-Kumar 2001) on women's experiences of reproduction in Jaipur, in communities living on the outskirts of Jaipur city. She noted that most women there regarded menstruation as a flow of waste or dirt, and were using menstrual cloths that had to be washed out of sight and hidden in cracks of stone or placed under other clothes to dry. Notions of shame and impurity thus combined in shaping women's menstrual practices and personal hygiene. Many poor women and girls in slums have no access to safe, clean toilets with water supplies.

According to the baseline survey carried out by the NGO Centre for Advocacy and Research (CFAR) in 2012 covering 236 households in seven urban slums of Jaipur, only 51.27 per cent of households had personal toilets in their homes. The availability of common public toilets was poor (CFAR 2012, 8). In addition, user charges also deterred people from using them; 47.46 per cent of households practised open defecation (*ibid.*).

In July 2015, the State Government of Rajasthan launched a free sanitary napkin distribution scheme called UDAAN, which replaced an earlier programme initiated in 2011–12 in select districts by the central Government of India.[5] In July 2015, the UDAAN scheme was started in Jaipur. The aim was that around 2 million girls, both school going and non-school going and 233,000 girls from slum areas were to be covered (Rajagopal *et al.* 2016).

Though UDAAN was primarily mandated for rural areas, the decision to include urban girls was largely influenced by constant advocacy by the NGO CFAR, working on issues related to WASH in urban slums of Jaipur. CFAR has been working in these slums since 2009. It has worked at multiple levels for crystallising the demands of the community, and making government service providers more responsive towards the needs of the urban poor.

CFAR (2015) published a study of unmet WASH and menstrual needs of pupils in 105 government schools. It showed many girls found it difficult to attend classes, went home from school, were sent home by staff, or dropped out of school altogether after menstruation began. They often experienced acute embarrassment, a sense of shame, and low self-esteem (CFAR 2015). Some manufacturers of sanitary pads were distributing their products on a charitable basis in schools, as a marketing and promotional exercise. However, this distribution was not carried out on a regular basis.

When the UDAAN scheme was launched in Jaipur, 200 girls from government schools and 70 girls from slum areas in Jaipur were provided with a three-month stock of sanitary pads. Each packet contained eight pads. In the first phase 50,000 pads were supplied. By 5 November 2015, around 45,500 napkins had been distributed to 15,000 girls – 12,500 school-going girls and 2,500 girls residing in slums (personal communication with officials in the Department of Health and Family Welfare, Government of Rajasthan, April 2016). The scheme was to be further expanded in a phased manner to seven districts by 2 October 2015 and to all districts by 8 March 2016 (*ibid.*). The distribution was carried out in the months of July to September 2015, via schools and at *Anganwari*[6] Centres.

Our research: purpose, methods, and participants

In April 2016, we undertook a study of the impact of UDAAN at the request of CFAR, which was written up as a report (Rajagopal *et al.* 2016). The objective was to measure the impact of the intervention on girls living in areas with few basic services, especially urban slums. It also aimed to assess both the direct and indirect benefits to girls in schools and the slums of Jaipur where CFAR works. As feminist researchers located in a social science research institute, this study provided us with an opportunity to engage with a subject that was critical to the empowerment of adolescent girls. The findings of the study could also be used to bring the subject centre-stage within policy discourse. CFAR was also keen on using this assessment as an advocacy tool, for influencing the state government to include urban girls in its coverage.

The study was carried out from April to June 2016. It involved a total of 270 girls (130 school-going and 140 non-school-going girls) in 12 slums in Jaipur, and within five government schools where the UDAAN pads had been directly distributed by the manufacturer. It covered girls in the age group of 10–20 years. The group was predominantly Hindu, and belonged to socially disadvantaged caste groups. Even though the scheme had been so short-lived, research could shed light on the wider issues around menstruation and the provision of sanitary pads to urban girls, including the knowledge and practices of girls around menstruation, the role of teachers and health providers, and the attitudes of mothers.

We used mixed research methods. Quantitative data were collected through a survey tool. Qualitative data were gathered through focus group discussions (FGDs) and indepth interviews. We visited schools for the research and also focused on non-schoolgoing girls in the slum areas, who were identified with the support of CFAR. An effort was made to facilitate an environment where the girls could talk openly about menstrual health and share their experiences.

Most of the girls in our research came from low-income households, where selfemployment was the main occupation. Parents were largely involved in petty trading and casual labour. Fathers drove auto-rickshaws, or did tailoring or gem polishing. Typical tasks for mothers included bangle-making, vegetable-vending, embroidery, and paper-bag making. About 15 per cent of the school-going girls helped out with these activities when they were not in school.

Twenty-three per cent of the non-school-going girls were also involved in various home-based economic activities like bangle-making, making paper bags, and embroidery work; a small proportion of girls were working as domestic help and a few were working in the formal sector such as export houses. All girls assisted their mothers with unpaid care work for the family.

The highest proportion of school-going girls (47 per cent) in our research belonged to Scheduled Caste[7] households, while the remainder of school-going girls were from General Caste[8] groups (27 per cent), Other Backward Castes (24.6 per cent), and Scheduled Tribe (1.5 per cent). In contrast, among non-school-going girls, the highest proportion were from General Caste groups (41.4 per cent), while the others were from Scheduled Caste (38 per cent), Other Backward Castes (15.7 per cent) and Scheduled Tribe (5.0 per cent).

The presence of more Scheduled Caste girls in schools corroborates the fact that government schools continue to be the mainstay institutions for children from disadvantaged communities. However, the higher proportion of non-school-going girls from the General Caste groups also indicates that despite having a better social status, the girls are often compelled to drop out of the school due to several social reasons.

The educational levels of parents were not high. Nearly half (48 per cent) of fathers of schoolgoing girls had attained education beyond secondary schooling, leaving after Grade 10, and only 18.1 per cent had never attended school. In contrast, 58 per cent fathers of non-schoolgoing girls had never attended school, and 16 per cent had attained Grade 10. A high proportion of mothers (70 per cent) did not have any formal education. Ninety-one per cent of mothers of non-school-going girls were not literate, compared with 63 per cent of mothers of school-going girls. The poor educational levels of mothers are significant in terms of the information shared by them on menstruation and related issues with their daughters.

In the following sections, we share some of the most interesting and important findings from the study. The concluding section posits the way forward for policy advocacy.

Awareness and sources of information regarding menstruation

Locally, the most common terms used by girls to refer to menstruation was 'period' (in English) and 'MC' (again referring to an English term, 'monthly cycle'). Most girls reported first menstruation between the ages of 10 and 15.

Three-quarters of school-going girls (73.3 per cent) and an even higher proportion of non-school-going girls reported not having any prior information regarding the onset of the menstrual cycle. This confirms earlier studies (Khanna *et al.* 2005; Sahayog 2016). They were totally unprepared for menstruation. During FGDs in government schools and the slum areas, one of the participants stated:

> I had no information regarding menstruation before I started my periods. I had only observed that on certain days, my mother did not enter the kitchen and cook. When I asked my mother about this, she did not given any reason or explanation. (Meena 16 years, during FGD with school-going girls in Jaipur city, June 2016)

All girls agreed that when they started their periods, the first person they went to was their mother. The role of schools in providing information (which could happen via teachers, media, or books) was negligible. Media outside school also had a negligible role. The lack of school attempts to discuss menstruation, including how to cope with periods in terms of hygiene, was a serious concern. During FGDs in schools, typical comments were:

> The teachers themselves are inhibited and do not discuss the topic openly. (Meenakshi, 15 years)

> When my friend started menstruating in the school, I was scared and embarrassed to see blood spots on her clothes. (Sunita, 16 years)

> The teacher asked me to go home and talk to my mother. (Reshma, 16 years)

Taboos, myths, and restrictions during menstruation

The taboos and myths associated with menstruation are pervasive, and continue to restrict women's and girls' participation in private and public spheres. Since menarche indicates puberty, sexual maturation, and consequent ability to reproduce, there is an anxiety around the sexuality of girls, and various restrictions are placed on their mobility.

It is significant to note that 88 per cent of all school-going and non-school-going girls had a negative feeling about menstruation, and considered menstrual blood as *ganda* (that is, unclean or impure). The biological purpose of menstruation in the female reproductive cycle was not widely understood. Instead, the common perceptions articulated were that body heat is thrown out during menstruation, and menstrual blood is the accumulated dirt that flows out of the body every month.

The deeply ingrained notions of ritual pollution and impurity associated with menstruation translate into taboos, myths, and euphemisms around menstruation. The restrictions placed on girls intensify during religious activities and occasions. Taboos and restrictions during menstruation included:

- Girls are not allowed to enter the kitchen to cook as they are regarded as 'impure' and cannot touch certain food items like *achaar* (pickle), as there is a widespread belief that preserved food items spoil. An associated belief is that eating hot and spicy food increases the flow of blood and hence there is a restriction on eating such food.
- Menstruating girls are not allowed to touch the *matka* (water pot).
- Participation in religious activities and performing religious rituals is strictly prohibited.
- Girls are not allowed to visit a temple or perform *pooja* (prayer); reading the Koran and offering *Namaz* (prayer) is also forbidden.
- Unmarried girls cannot serve food to fathers and brothers during menstruation.
- Girls did not wash their hair for three days during their periods and could enter the temple or place of worship at home and kitchen thereafter (field notes, June 2016).

Other possible restrictions on mobility and carrying out household chores like sweeping, and washing clothes and utensils did not emerge as a significant factor in the study. However, the practical implications of leaving home without sanitary protection that could be relied on were clear, and as stated earlier, the central focus of the study.

Usage of sanitary protection and problems in disposal

Importantly, a major inter-generational change was observed, related to use of modern forms of sanitary protection. Common terms used to refer to sanitary pads were pads or brand names like Whisper or Carefree.

Nearly three-quarters (73 per cent) of both school-going and non-school-going girls used sanitary pads as protection during menstruation. The use of sanitary pads was found to be higher among school-going girls than non-school-going girls. The use of cloth was comparatively higher among non-school-going girls.

During the FGDs, girls from both groups said they often combined use of cloth and sanitary pads. The out-of-school girls in the slums, especially those from poorer backgrounds, said when they did not have money to buy pads, they had no choice but to revert to using cloth. The commonly used commercial brand was Whisper or Carefree. The research team was informed that these products have also been distributed in schools free of cost by the company. These distributions happened before UDAAN and have continued to happen afterwards. Given the main aim of the UDAAN programme was to make available sanitary pads on a regular basis free of costs, it was felt that it would help change practice especially for girls who could not afford to buy commercial pads.

The majority of girls who have used sanitary pads reported that they change the pads twice a day as they felt that not doing so would lead to infection. However, this was sometimes impossible due to the lack of availability of clean washrooms/toilets both within homes and in schools. Girls in a government school said:

> If we go to school during periods we have to use the toilet at least once to change napkins. (Karishma, 17 years, FGD, May 2016)

> The toilets are not clean. In such a situation we try and avoid using the toilets. We also refrain from drinking too much water. (Dikshita, 16 years, FGD, May 2016)

The girls who used cloths reported various problems in cleaning, washing, and drying the cloth. Eighteen per cent of those who used cloths reported they dried them under other garments. The remaining 40 per cent reported they dry cloths in a secluded area away from the gaze of the male members of the family. Field observations revealed most houses in the slum areas are located in congested lanes. The laundry was mostly washed outside the homes in the lanes, and girls found it almost impossible to wash and dry the cloth used for menstruation publicly.

An essential aspect of menstrual hygiene and management is disposal of used pads. The lack of appropriate disposal mechanisms is a serious problem. The majority of girls reported that they wrapped the napkins in a newspaper or put them in plastic bags before disposing of them. The disposal was done under cover and girls said that they feel extremely embarrassed if someone watched them disposing of the used pads. The lack of hygienic public disposal systems is acute in the slum areas.

Problems faced during menstruation

Health problems

Numerous problems were reported by both school-going and non-school-going girls during menstruation. A high proportion of girls reported suffering from abdominal cramps, body ache, and weakness. Nausea and vomiting during menstruation was also common. A small percentage resorted to home remedies. Forty-five per cent of girls also reported having itching and burning and swelling in the vagina, leucorrhoea and dysmenorrhoea. Girls using cloths also stated that usage of cloth led to laceration and discomfort. Most girls did not take any medication for these problems or consult a doctor. The inadequacy of health services within reach is also a contributing factor.

School attendance problems

Several factors impact regular attendance and continuation of girls in schools in Rajasthan. These include proximity of schools from home, especially secondary schools, presence of women teachers in schools, quality of teaching and learning, and availability of infrastructure facilities including toilets/restrooms/common rooms. In addition, girl's attendance is also influenced by unmet menstrual needs.

While a high proportion of girls (83.8 per cent) reported that they attended school during menstruation, physical management of menstruation was a problem. The problems encountered include: unhygienic toilets due to lack of running water; and the dearth of covered dustbins compels girls to throw the used napkins inside the toilets, clogging them and making them unusable. Besides, there is no soap in the toilets for washing. The girls also hesitate to ask for sanitary napkins from teachers. In co-educational schools girls find it difficult to carry and change sanitary napkins for fear of being teased by boys.

Many girls stated missing school for a day or two due to abdominal cramps and pain. They also stated that they have to travel by public transport and often do not get a seat on the bus and have to stand for long durations. The discussions with school teachers also highlighted this fact.

The lack of forums in schools where girls and boys can discuss issues related to menstrual health and hygiene emerged as a critical gap. The low levels of information regarding menstrual processes and the continuation of notions of pollution and impurity points to the inadequacy of the schooling system to address this issue. This is further compounded by the culture of silence around menstruation within homes contributing to a negative feeling about a natural biological process. It is also evident that school curricula have failed to address the existing misconceptions and taboos around menstruation.

Girls' experience of UDAAN

All the school-going girls in the sample had received sanitary napkins in their schools; 70 per cent of them also reported that a few instructions on usage and disposal were given at the time of distribution. However, in each school the distribution pattern differed. A higher proportion of girls (41.6 per cent) reported that they had received the sanitary napkins three times, 36.1 per cent of girls said they had got the sanitary napkins only once, and 22.3 per cent of girls reported they had received the sanitary napkins twice. The majority reported that the sanitary napkins lasted only for two months; for those who shared the napkins with other female members in the family, the packets lasted only for one menstrual cycle.

A high proportion of non-school-going girls in the slums were aware of the UDAAN scheme. They stated being given information regarding the usage and disposal of sanitary napkins during meetings organised by CFAR. Each girl was given a set of three packets. However, the distribution was carried out only once; 65 per cent of non-school-going girls had used the packets themselves; but 35 per cent of girls reported that they had also shared the napkins with their mothers and sisters. The majority of girls said that the three packets lasted for two months.

> The meetings with the adolescent girls are organised twice a week every Monday and Friday. Inputs are also provided by CFAR team to girls during these meetings. The main issues discussed are sanitation and hygiene, menstrual hygiene, nutrition, and health. All girls in the age group of 11–18 years were given the napkins in the month of September 2015. A total of 160 girls benefited from the Udaan scheme. Three packets were given to each girl. Even today about 10 per cent of girls in the slums use cloth, as they cannot afford to buy sanitary napkins. (FGD with Accredited Social Health Activist (ASHA) and Mahila Arogya Samiti (MAS) members, June 2016)[9]

Eighty-three per cent of school-going girls reported that even though the distribution of free napkins was erratic, they continued to use sanitary napkins. However, 17 per cent of girls also reported they had gone back to using cloth during menstruation as they could not afford to buy napkins on a regular basis. Fifty-three per cent of girls who were continuing to use napkins reported that they were spending up to Rs 50 per month, 10 per cent of girls were spending up to Rs 75 and 22 per cent of girls stated spending more than Rs 75 per month on purchasing napkins.

The co-ordinators in schools reported that since the distribution had been irregular, they were not able to respond or give a definitive answer to the girls regarding the supply of the next lot of sanitary napkins.

Almost all the school-going and non-school-going girls felt that the UDAAN scheme had benefited them and helped save money. It also saved them the effort of purchasing sanitary napkins from the market (girls continue to be inhibited in asking for a packet of sanitary napkins over the counter). They expressed a willingness to purchase the napkins at a subsidised rate, but demanded that the supply in school be regularised.

A two-thirds majority of non-school-going girls (67 per cent) said after the distribution, they had started using sanitary napkins more regularly. The free supply of UDAAN napkins had helped in saving money. However, girls who discontinued usage said that the free packets finished in two months and they could not afford to buy sanitary napkins on a regular basis from the market.

> I have four daughters and all of them have their monthly cycles. I cannot afford to buy napkins; so I tell them to use cloth. I know it is not hygienic as I have suffered due to infection myself but I have little choice. (Interview with a mother in a slum area, May 2016)

The ASHA and MAS members also felt that the UDAAN scheme had helped girls, but since the napkins were distributed only once, many girls had to discontinue usage. They recommended that this programme should be continued and monitored closely.

Several suggestions were put forth by girls (both in school and in slums) regarding the free napkins scheme. These included:

- Government should ensure regular/monthly supply of good-quality sanitary pads to all school-going and non-school-going girls in urban and rural areas.
- Sanitary napkins should be made available at the *Anganwari* centres at a nominal rate.
- Information regarding menstruation, related problems, and usage of sanitary napkins should be given to all girls in school and in the slum areas.

Discussion

To us, it is evident that the free distribution of napkins scheme has benefited a number of girls in urban areas of Jaipur city. The fact that sanitary napkins were made available in the school and in the slum areas made it convenient for girls as they did not have to source it from the market. For the non-users it helped to change practice to some extent, though they reverted to using cloth due to irregular supply of napkins. The overall suggestions given by the girls focus on the need for a regular supply of napkins in schools and slum areas, as well as initiating discussions on menstrual health and hygiene.

In a context where girls face multiple disadvantages and scarce resources, a focus on menstrual health and management is important. The insights gained from our research point to the fact that while providing physical and material means for menstrual management is crucial, it does not necessarily empower girls who lack basic information about their bodies. Such knowledge is critical if girls are to feel confident about normal bodily changes and attain a sense of positive body awareness (Kirk and Sommer 2006). The need for a holistic response in creating gender-friendly initiatives and promoting awareness on health and hygiene to address puberty and menstruation challenges also emerges as critical.

A discernible inter-generational change in usage of commercially produced sanitary protection was observed. However, the silence around menstruation, compounded by the lack of information regarding bodily processes, the adherence to patriarchal beliefs and taboos, and the lack of questioning by the girls, are serious concerns that need to be addressed at various levels.

Given the gender gap in school enrolment and attendance at higher stages of schooling in the state, disruption in school attendance during menstruation is worrisome. Poor sanitary facilities and non-availability of clean toilets with water in schools make it unsuitable for changing sanitary pads and for disposing of menstrual waste. This situation discourages girls from attending school. Further poor protection and inadequate washing facilities increase susceptibility to infection and related problems.

School curricula typically do not cover the topic of sexual maturation and onset of menarche in a gender-friendly manner. It does not help girls and boys to understand the changes occurring in their bodies. Though the text-books focus on the biological and technical aspects of human reproduction, no effort is made to discuss the social and emotional aspects which the adolescents need to understand. The crucial role of teachers and the need for open discussions and dialogues within the schooling environment is selfevident.

While the findings highlight the positive impact of the UDAAN scheme, any programming around the issue of menstrual hygiene management should be based on an in-depth analysis of both urban and rural contexts. Provisioning of sanitary protection is a useful response, but only part of a solution. Several other mechanisms need to be in place to enable girls to manage menstruation with confidence and dignity. Also, governmentinitiated schemes that promote change in practice are rendered meaningless unless they can be sustained over a period of time. When we probed further on why distribution under UDAAN had been discontinued, we did not get a satisfactory response from the government officials. It is evident that the officials had not done any long-term planning or allocated adequate budget to cover urban areas.

Conclusion

More research is required to map interventions that are contextually designed and address multiple challenges of unmet menstrual needs faced by adolescents. Menstrual hygiene is an important element in this, but is not the only issue in a context in which puberty, sexuality, and sexual and reproductive health are not discussed fully and openly in families, communities, or schools. A well-informed continuous school education and empowerment programme for boys and girls needs to be initiated to minimise stigma around menstruation. Encouraging adolescent forums to help shape healthy menstrual attitudes also emerges as critical. Engaging with men and boys on these issues, including menstruation, is crucial. NGOs and civil society organisations can take a lead in initiating these dialogues and interventions at various levels.

Bearing in mind its effect on reducing girls' confidence and freedom to attend school and generally move around freely in the community, the issue of menstrual hygiene management needs to be brought centre stage within policy discourse as issues of body awareness are critical to adolescent empowerment. Menstrual hygiene needs to be addressed comprehensively, to give women and girls the confidence and space to voice their need for improved menstrual hygiene. A multi-sectoral approach is essential to help break the silence on the issue by leveraging and converging with different government schemes across key sectors, including WASH, reproductive health, education, and rights, to reach out systematically to adolescent girls and boys with relevant information. NGOs like CFAR can play an important part in advocacy and research, as well as community interventions. Another priority area of work is continuous and systematic engagement and capacity building of frontline workers like *Anganwari* workers, ASHA, and teachers is essential to promote understanding on issues related to menstruation and menstrual hygiene management.

In the context of the UDAAN scheme specifically, there is an urgent need to streamline guidelines and put monitoring mechanisms in place for making it effective. The continued and regular supply of napkins is crucial to support a change in practice among non-users. Critically, the issue is one of poverty, and partnerships could be developed with the many groups producing low-cost sanitary napkins in the state. Given the demand and inability of many girls to source napkins from the market, the opportunity lies in linking up with these groups for universal coverage.

Notes

1. The use of the term 'menstrual hygiene' presents the issue of menstruation in the terms of technical approaches to WASH, but is limited to dealing with the practicalities. Some feminist activists highlight that without working to challenge social norms about menstruation, stigma will persist for a natural biological function of healthy women, which is not unclean or impure.
2. 'Sanitary napkin' is a formal and old-fashioned term which does not describe the products of today offered to women – which are pads, not cloths. However, within government officials use the word napkins. Most women refer to them using brand names, e.g. Whisper.
3. For details, see www.jatansansthan.org and www.vishakhawe.org (last checked 24 May 2017).
4. The link between unmet needs for menstrual hygiene and reproductive tract infections in India is still being researched, and more studies are needed (Anand *et al.* 2015). However, a media report by a female reporter in a local newspaper, about district hospitals in Rajasthan, estimated that around 50 per cent of the female outpatient cases she had encountered had reproductive tract infections, and to a significant extent she considered these attributable to poor hygiene practices during menstruation (Dainik Bhaskar 2015).
5. In 2011–12, the Menstrual Hygiene Programme was initiated in selected districts of Rajasthan under the National Rural Health Mission (NRHM) of the Government of India. The scheme reached out to rural girls in the age group of 10–19 years. Under the scheme, a packet of six sanitary napkins were sold to the girls at the cost of Rs 6 per packet by the local Accredited Social Health Activist (ASHA). ASHA are designated community health workers instituted by the Government of India's Ministry of Health and Family Welfare as part of the NRHM. In 2014–15, the Government of India approved the expansion of this programme to 16 districts in the state, and rural girls were to be supplied with sanitary napkins. In 2015–16, the number of districts was reduced from 16 to 12.
6. *Anganwari* (courtyard) centres are part of the Integrated Child Development Scheme of the Government of India to address issues related to development of children in the age group 3–6 years.
7. Scheduled Castes are the officially designated disadvantaged communities in India that have been accorded special status by the Constitution of India.

8. General Castes or Forward Castes is a term used in India for the upper caste groups who are considered socially, educationally, and economically advanced. These groups of people do not qualify for any of the affirmative action schemes operated by the Government of India.
9. Mahila Arogya Samitis are constituted as part of the National Urban Health Mission in each slum area to facilitate linkages to community health services.

Notes on contributors

Shobhita Rajagopal is Associate Professor at the Institute of Development Studies, Jaipur. Email: shobhita@idsj.org

Kanchan Mathur is Professor at the Institute of Development Studies, Jaipur. Email: kanchan@idsj.org

References

Anand, Enu, Jayakant Singh and Sayeed Unisa (2015) 'Menstrual hygiene practices and its association with reproductive tract infections and abnormal vaginal discharge among women in India', *Sexual & Reproductive Healthcare* 6(4): 249–54

Centre for Advocacy and Research (2012) *Baseline Survey of Select Slums of Jaipur*, Jaipur: CFAR

Centre for Advocacy and Research (2015) *Status of Health, Sanitation and Hygiene in Government Schools of Jaipur: A Study of 105 Government Schools*, New Delhi: CFAR

Dainik Bhaskar (2015) 'Sanitary napkin na Milne se, rajya ki ek crore mahilayein sankraman ki shikar', Jaipur, 25 May

Dube, Shubha and Kirti Sharma (2012) 'Knowledge, attitude and practice regarding reproductive health among urban and rural girls: a comparative study', *Ethno Med* 6(2): 85–94, www.krepublishers.com (last checked 1 June 2016)

Government of India (2015) *Menstrual Hygiene Management: National Guidelines, Ministry of Drinking Water and Sanitation*, New Delhi: Government of India

Government of India (2016) 'Revised Guidelines for Menstrual Hygiene Scheme', Ministry of Health and Family Welfare, http://nhm.gov.in/nrhm-updates/522-revised guidelines (last checked 19 June 2017)

Government of Rajasthan (2016) *Economic Survey-2015-16*, Rajasthan: Directorate of Economics and Statistics, Department of Planning

Government of Rajasthan (2017) *State Strategy and Action Plan for Prevention of Child Marriage: Towards creating a child marriage free Rajasthan*, Jaipur: Government of Rajasthan

Khanna, Anoop, R.S Goyal and Rahul Bhawsar (2005) 'Menstrual practices and reproductive problems: a study of adolescent girls in Rajasthan', *Journal of Health Management* 7(91): 91–107

Kirk, Jackie and Marni Sommer (2006) *Menstruation and Body Awareness: Linking Girls' Health with Girls Education*, Royal Tropical Institute (KIT) Special on Gender and Health, Amsterdam: KIT, http://www.susana.org/en/resources/library/details/1200 (last checked 19 June 2017)

National Family Health Survey (2015-16) 'Fact sheet for key indicators', http://rchiips.org/NFHS/factsheet_NFHS-4.shtml, (last checked 19 June 2017)

Niti Aayog (National Institution for Transforming India) (2017) 'Maternal Mortality', http://niti.gov.in/content/maternal-mortality-ratio-mmr-100000-live-births (last checked 19 June 2017)

Population Foundation of India (PFI) (2012) *Facts and Factors: State of Inclusive WATSAN in cities,* 01 Jaipur, New Delhi: PFI

Rajagopal, Shobita and R.S. Sharma (2016) *Open and Distance Learning as a Cost Effective Option for Secondary Level Schooling in India: Potential and Prerequisites in Rajasthan: A Research Report,* Jaipur: Institute of Development Studies

Rajagopal, Shobita, Kanchan Mathur and R.S. Sharma (2016) *Menstrual Hygiene Management Intervention in Jaipur: An Impact Assessment,* Jaipur: Institute of Development Studies

Sahayog (2016) *Local Beliefs and Practices Around Menstruation: A Qualitative Study in Selected Blocks of Three Districts in Uttar Pradesh and one District in Uttarakhand,* Lucknow: Sahayog

U-DISE (Unified District Information System for Education) 2014-15 (2015) www.dise.in (last checked 19 June 2017)

Unnithan-Kumar, Maya (2001) 'Emotion, agency and access to healthcare: women's experiences of reproduction in Jaipur', in Soraya Tremayne (ed.) *Managing Reproductive Life: Cross-Cultural Themes in Sexuality and Fertility. Fertility, Reproduction, and Sexuality,* Oxford: Berghahn Books, 27–51

Resources

Compiled by Liz Cooke

Gender and WASH (water, sanitation and hygiene): Policy

Women and WASH: Water, Sanitation and Hygiene for Women's Rights and Gender Equality, Briefing Note (2013) Shamila Jansz and Jane Wilbur, WaterAid, https://washmatters.wateraid.org/publications, (last accessed 17 September 2019), 4 pp.

This short paper provides a useful and accessible introduction to the topic of gender and WASH. Outlining the key focus areas for a gendered approach to WASH, the issues covered are: maternal and newborn health; girls' education; menstrual hygiene; violence against women; dignity and self-esteem; inequality and discrimination; economic empowerment; and women's rights. The paper ends with a short case study from India, describing a successful project which supported women to demand better services from their water provider, resulting in an average 20 per cent less time spent collecting water.

We Can't Wait: A Report on Sanitation and Hygiene for Women and Girls (2013) Domestos, WaterAid, and WSSCC, https://washmatters.wateraid.org/publications/we-cant-wait-a-report-on-sanitation-and-hygiene-for-women-and-girls, (last accessed 17 September 2019) 27 pp.

Another helpful introduction to the topic, this paper was published in 2013 by multinational company Unilever, in conjunction with the international NGO WaterAid, and the United Nations-hosted Water Supply and Sanitation Collaborative Council as part of advocacy around the inauguration of International World Toilet Day. The paper outlines the scale of what it terms 'the global sanitation crisis', and what it means for women and girls, in particular, touching on areas such as (lack of) menstrual hygiene at home, school, and in the workplace, and the risk of ill health, shame, harassment, and violence when open defecation is the only option in the absence of safe, hygienic toilets. The paper includes useful facts and figures, and (in brief) the voices of some of those struggling to live with inadequate water and sanitation. Unsurprisingly, given that the paper comes from Unilever, there is a section on the roles the private sector can play in improving sanitation, through

http://dx.doi.org/10.3362/9781788530866.011

public–private partnerships, direct service delivery, and as advocates in countries for improved governance, financing, and capacity-building (making the point that it is national governments who are the duty bearers when it comes to the Human Right to Water and Sanitation). Final recommendations for what should be included in any forthcoming Sustainable Development Goal (SDG) on water and sanitation (the paper was published in 2013), can be compared with what was ultimately decided on for inclusion in SDG 6, in 2016.

Achieving Gender Equality Through WASH: GADN Briefing (2016) Kate Bishop, London: Gender & Development Network (GADN), https:// static1.squarespace.com/static/536c4ee8e4b0b60bc6ca7c74/t/56f41cee2fe 131a7e0b9651c/1458838767309/Achieving+gender+equality+through+ WASH+-+April+2016.pdf (last accessed 17 September 2019), 18 pp.

This briefing paper, published by GADN partnered with WaterAid, shows that equitable and universal access cannot be achieved without specific gender equality measures in WASH policy and programming to ensure that the rights of girls and women to water and sanitation are met. The aim of the briefing is to set out the multiple links between gender equality and WASH to encourage dialogue, mutual understanding, and consensus between gender equality and WASH policymakers and practitioners. Ideally, a more detailed examination of the linkages through new research and innovative programme development will be carried out as a result.

'Swimming upstream: why sanitation, hygiene and water are so important to mothers and their daughters' (2010) Clarissa Brocklehurst and Jamie Bartram, Bulletin of the World Health Organization 88(7): 482–82, www.who.int/bulletin/volumes/88/7/10-080077.pdf?ua=1 (last accessed 19 September 2019)

In this short piece, the authors describe the inter-generational effects for women and girls of inadequate WASH. Starting with problems around water collection during pregnancy, the risks to infant health from diarrhoea, a vicious cycle contributes to keeping women in ill health, out of education, in poverty, and bearing sickly children.

Insecurity and Indignity: Women's Experiences in the Slums of Nairobi, Kenya (2010) Amnesty International, London: Amnesty International Publications, www. amnesty.org/en/documents/AFR32/002/2010/en/, (last accessed 17 September 2019), 59 pp.

This report illustrates the realities of life for women in slums and informal settlements, who must contend with inadequate public services, including provision of safe and clean water and sanitation, and high levels of insecurity and violence. The report gathered evidence in four informal settlements in Nairobi, and Chapter 5, 'Women's Lack of Safety and Access to Essential

Services', details the lived experiences of individual women and girls who lack adequate access to toilets and bathing facilities. Crucial issues were health and privacy, and violence against women.

Report of the Special Rapporteur on the Human Right to Safe Drinking Water and Sanitation (A/HRC/33/49) (2016) The United Nations General Assembly, https://www.refworld.org/docid/57cd86474.html (last accessed 19 September 2019), 21 pp.

The UN Resolution on the Human Right to Water and Sanitation (see below) calls for an annual report from an independent expert – the Special Rapporteur on the human rights to safe drinking water and sanitation – to be submitted to the UN General Assembly. In 2016, the Rapporteur's report focused on gender equality in the realisation of the human rights to water and sanitation. The 21-page report includes discussion on gender equality in law and policies; intersectionality and multiple forms of discrimination; harmful social norms, stigma, and stereotypes; gender-based violence and psychosocial stress; availability and affordability; participation; empowerment; and accountability. The report argues that efforts to overcome gender inequality in respect of the right to water and sanitation must address women's strategic needs, such as the eradication of harmful gender stereotypes, together with practical interventions focusing on meeting women's material needs, e.g. adequate menstrual hygiene facilities. A leaflet summarising the key issues and challenges contained in the report (and presented in a more user-friendly style than the rather off-putting, formal report!) is available at www.ohchr.org/Documents/Issues/Water/Pamplet_GenderEquality.pdf   (last   accessed 19 September 2019), 2 pp.

Sustainable Development Goal 6: Ensure Access to Water and Sanitation for All, www.un.org/sustainabledevelopment/water-and-sanitation/ (last accessed 17 September 2019)

SDG 6 – ensuring access to water and sanitation for all – builds on Millennium Development Goal Target 7c, which was to halve by 2015 the number of people without access to safe drinking water and basic sanitation. The drinking water MDG target was met by 2015, but not that of sanitation. SDG 6 represents the international community's aim of 'achiev [ing] universal and equitable access to safe and affordable drinking water for all' by 2030. Of the eight specific targets for SDG 6, only target two makes explicit reference to gender issues, with a stated aim of 'achiev[ing] access to adequate and equitable sanitation and hygiene for all and end open defecation, paying special attention to the needs of women and girls in those vulnerable situations', and there are no explicit gender indicators included, either against this target or any others. A full list of SDG 6 targets, indicators, and further information can be found at the link above.

The Human Right to Water and Sanitation (2010) The United Nations General Assembly, https://digitallibrary.un.org/record/687002 (last accessed 17 September 2019), 3 pp.

While the right to water and sanitation has been included in previous United Nations (UN) conventions, covenants, resolutions, and reports, in July 2010 the right to safe and clean water and sanitation as a human right was made explicit in this stand-alone resolution from the UN General Assembly (Resolution A/RES/64/292). A 38-page UN factsheet, *The Right to Water* (2010), provides much useful information, see www.ohchr.org/Documents/Publications/FactSheet35en.pdf (last accessed 17 September 2019), and a four-page timeline of milestones on the road to the 2010 Resolution can be found at www.un.org/waterforlifedecade/pdf/human_right_to_water_and_sanitation_milestones.pdf (last accessed 19 September 2019).

Equity and Inclusion: A Rights-based Approach (2010) Louisa Gosling, London: WaterAid, https://resourcecentre.savethechildren.net/node/6371/pdf/6371.pdf (last accessed 17 September 2019), 36 pp.

Designed by international NGO WaterAid to guide its own work on WASH, the Equity and Inclusion Framework set out in this report has become highly influential in the sector as a whole. The Framework first sets out WaterAid's position and approach – defining the principles of equity and inclusion as they relate to WASH, and the application of them through the adoption of an anti-poverty, rights-based (rather than needs-based) focus, working to include the most disadvantaged people (who may include women, people with disabilities, minority ethnic groups, and people belonging to specific castes, for example) and being aware of the dynamics that cause discrimination, marginalisation, and exclusion at family, community, national, and international levels. The approach requires an understanding of why people lack access to adequate WASH, a commitment to working with duty bearers to strengthen their capacity to deliver, and a commitment to support those without adequate provision to claim their rights to WASH. The Framework goes on to provide standards and indicators for equity and inclusion, an explanation of terms, and examples of marginalised groups in relation to WASH.

Water and Sanitation for Disabled People and Other Vulnerable Groups: Designing Services to Improve Accessibility (2005) Hazel Jones and Bob Reed, Loughborough: Water, Engineering and Development Centre (WEDC), ISBN: 9781843800798, see https://wedc-knowledge.lboro.ac.uk/details.html?id=16357 (last accessed 17 September 2019), 322 pp.

Following the recognition that women's specific needs were routinely being ignored in WASH provision, this path-breaking work, published in 2005, sought to extend inclusion in domestic WASH programmes to the hitherto largely ignored demographic of people with disabilities, along with others such as elderly people, pregnant women, and people living with illness. Written for WASH planners and those working on the ground to provide services, the book has a strong practical focus, combining discussion of disability and WASH, programming advice, and technical design advice.

Leave No One Behind: Voices of Women, Adolescent Girls, Elderly and Disabled People, and Sanitation Workers (2015) Water Supply and Sanitation Collaborative Council (WSSCC) and Freshwater Action Network South Asia (FANSA), http://wsscc.org/resources-feed/leave-no-one-behind-voices-of-women-adolescent-girls-elderlypersons-with-disabilities-and-sanitation-workforce/ (last accessed 17 September 2019), 40 pp.

This advocacy report published by the WSSCC and the FANSA, was produced for the South Asian Conference on Sanitation (SACOSAN) VI in 2016. Aiming to bring to the voices of those 'who are barely visible; who rarely speak, decide or sign anything' (p. 7) to the attention of decision-makers at this regularly held ministerial conference, the report relates the experiences of those whose needs are being ignored, including sanitation workers and waste collectors. Based on the results of consultations with marginalised groups of people – including transgender communities, plantation workers, and fisherfolk – in Afghanistan, Bangladesh, Bhutan, India, Nepal, the Maldives, Pakistan, and Sri Lanka, the paper sets out a list of key demands (which include consultation with regard to the building of WASH facilities, and community ownership) plus a number of recommendations for bodies planning, designing, and delivering sanitation and hygiene projects and services.

Governance and accountability

Gender Practice in Water Governance Programmes: From Design to Results, WGF Report No. 4 (2014) Moa Cortobius and Marianne Kjellén, Stockholm: Stockholm International Water Institute, http://watergovernance.org/resources/genderpractice-in-water-governance-programmes-from-design-to-results/, (last accessed 17 September 2019), 30 pp.

This report assesses the strategies and results of 11 water and sanitation programmes – located in Central and Southern America, Eastern Europe, Africa, and the Pacific – that aimed to incorporate gender equality issues into their design. Arguing that despite the widely recognised importance of women's role in water management (both in the household and in small-scale agriculture), the strong engineering focus of many water and sanitation programmes means integrating social concerns, particularly around gender, is challenging. Key findings of the report include the need for genuine commitment to the goal of gender mainstreaming on the part of programme leadership, and the willingness to bring in gender expertise, for example, through alliances with women's organisations. Further, agencies and organisations involved in water and sanitation governance need to review their own structures and practices, and also improve their understanding of the power dynamics that reinforce gender inequalities more broadly. An interesting point made by the authors is the emphasis in the programmes assessed on the improved efficiency and sustainability that would derive from adopting a gendered approach. Only one of the programmes examined justified its gender work in terms of promoting gender equality and the empowerment of women. This is in a context, as the authors explain, of increasing donor pressure to demonstrate cost-effectiveness and development discourse that emphasises economic and social benefits, rather than issues of justice or rights.

'Grassroots women's accountability mechanisms: strengthening urban governance through organising and partnerships' (2015) Rachael Wyant and Katarina Spasić, *Gender & Development* 23(1): 95–111, available at http:// policy-practice.oxfam.org.uk/publications/grassroots-womens-accountability-mechanisms-strengtheningurban-governance-thro-347213 (last accessed 19 September 2019)

This article details the experiences and lessons learned from an 18-month project undertaken by the grassroots women's network The Huairou Commission, which established women's groups to participate and monitor decision-making and basic service delivery in poor areas of the cities of Metro Manila in the Philippines, and Thankot in Nepal. The initiative was undertaken in the context of the trend towards decentralisation, which is often seen as a potential solution to the problem of poor governance and corruption, but where, the authors argue, community-driven, bottom-up strategies are needed to hold governments to account. The Nepal case study focuses specifically on women's action to improve access to drinking water and sanitation.

Oxfam Social Accountability and WASH Case Studies (2017) Social Accountability in Lebanon: Promoting Dialogue in Humanitarian and Development WASH Programmes, http://policy-practice.oxfam.org.uk/publications/social-accountabilityin-lebanon-promoting-dialogue-in-humanitarian-and-develop-620219 (last accessed 17 September 2019), 6 pp.

Social Accountability in Pakistan: Participatory Governance in Urban WASH, http:// policy-practice.oxfam.org.uk/publications/social-accountability-in-pakistan-participatory-governance-in-urban-wash-620222 (last accessed 17 September 2019), 8 pp.

Social Accountability in Sierra Leone: Influencing for Pro-poor WASH Investment in the 24-month Post-Ebola Recovery Planning, http://policy-practice.oxfam. org.uk/publications/social-accountability-in-sierra-leone-influencing-for-pro-poorwash-investment-620223 (last accessed 17 September 2019), 8 pp.

Social Accountability in Tajikistan: Enhancing Trust Between Communities and Water Service Providers, http://policy-practice.oxfam.org.uk/publications/socia-laccountability-in-tajikistan-enhancing-trust-between-communities-and-wat-620224 (last accessed 17 September 2019), 6 pp.

These case studies from some of Oxfam's social accountability and WASH projects outline experiences and key learning in a variety of contexts. They provide insight into the kind of work being undertaken by international NGOs to support citizen engagement with WASH provision and governance, and all include some reference to gender issues.

A Political Ecology of Women, Water and Global Environmental Change (2015) Stephanie Buechler and Anne-Marie S. Hanson (eds.), London and New York: Routledge, ISBN: 9781138232242

With a focus on environmental issues, this edited volume examines rural and urban livelihoods dependent on rivers, lakes, wetlands, and coastal locations, and illustrates the ways in which gender interacts with other social and geographical factors in water use, management, and governance. With case studies from Central and South Asia, Northern, Central and Southern Africa, and South and North America, the book makes clear the gendered nature of policies and practices around water management and climate change, water pollution, large-scale development and dams, water for agricultural use, and knowledge production, globally. Case studies also provide examples of women-led adaptation to pressure on water resources in the face of global environmental change.

Gender and WASH: Practice

Gender in Water and Sanitation (2010) The Water and Sanitation Program, Nairobi: WSP and World Bank, www.wsp.org/sites/wsp.org/files/publications/WSPgender-water-sanitation.pdf (last accessed 17 September 2019), 40 pp.

The Introduction to this paper makes clear the disproportionate effect on women and girls of inadequate WASH provision, and how this both causes and reinforces gender equality, and hampers countries' long-term economic development. Aimed at those working to mainstream gender in the sector – government ministries, NGOs, WASH providers, donors, etc. – the paper discusses adopting a gendered approach in policy; in WASH provision in the workplace, and urban and rural areas; in monitoring and evaluation; in civil society initiatives; in hygiene promotion; and in relation to WASH and HIV/AIDS. With checklists and examples of good practice accompanying each section, the paper is a practical guide for planning and reviewing gendered WASH responses across the sector.

Violence, Gender and Wash: A Practitioners Toolkit: Making Water, Santitation and Hygiene Safer Through Improved Programming and Services (2014), Sarah House,

Suzanne Ferron, Marni Sommer, and Sue Cavill, SHARE Consortium, http://violence-wash.lboro.ac.uk/ (last accessed 17 September 2019)

This comprehensive toolkit contains a wealth of information and practical materials designed to address the increased vulnerabilities that can arise from lack of access to adequate WASH services. Intended for use by WASH practitioners in development, humanitarian, and transitional contexts, it is also of value for those working on gender-based violence, gender, protection, health, and education. Content is organised into briefings on improving WASH programming in relation to violence; institutional commitment and staff capacity; and the protection sector and WASH. Eight tool sets provide, for example, methodologies on working with communities, case studies of violence, gender and WASH, and case studies of good practice in policy and programming. Because of the sheer volume of content, the toolkit takes a little bit of time to get to grips with in terms of its organisation. However, it is a resource of major importance to all those working to counter violence in the WASH sector and beyond.

Menstrual Hygiene Matters: A Resource for Improving Menstrual Hygiene Around the World (2012), Sarah House, Thérèse Mahon, and Sue Cavill, London: WaterAid, www.wateraid.org/what-we-do/our-approach/research-and-publications/viewpublication?id=02309d73-8e41-4d04-b2ef-6641f6616a4f (last accessed 17 September 2019)

Aimed at improving practices for women and girls in lowerand middle-income countries, *Menstrual Hygiene Matters* is a major resource not only for WASH practitioners, but for anyone wishing to gain a comprehensive understanding of the issue. Hugely informative and accessibly written and presented, it comprises nine modules, which cover key aspects of menstrual hygiene in different settings, including communities, schools, and emergencies. Each module is accompanied by its own toolkit, which includes checklists, technical guidance, case studies, further information, and a bibliography. It is downloadable as a single document, or as individual modules and toolkits.

Resource Guide. Working Effectively with Women and Men in Water, Sanitation and Hygiene Programs: Learnings from Research on Gender Outcomes from Rural Water, Sanitation and Hygiene Projects in Vanuatu and Fiji (2010), Gabrielle Halcrow, Claire Rowland, Juliet Willetts, Joanne Crawford, and Naomi Carrard, Sydney: International Women's Development Agency and Institute for Sustainable Futures, University of Technology Sydney, www.genderinpacificwash.info/system/resources/BAhbBlsHOgZmIj4yMDExLzAxLzI0LzE5LzA0LzI3LzIwMi9XQVNIX1JFU09VUkNFX0dVSURFX2ZpbmFsNHdlYi5wZGY/WASH%2520RESOURCE%2520GUIDE-final4web.pdf (last accessed 17 September 2019), 68 pp.

With a focus on Pacific Island countries, this is a resource aimed at WASH practitioners, to enable them to '[r]ecognise, plan for, support and monitor social outcomes for women and men as part of WASH projects' (p. 5). With a strong emphasis on community participation, this is essentially a short 'how to' guide to understanding and implementing gender mainstreaming in WASH programmes, which could perhaps equally be used for staff training in the area of gender and WASH. Indeed, Part 3 of the guide, 'People & Organisations', focuses on those implementing WASH programmes, and the importance of looking at attitudes, policies, and practices relating to gender equality within their own institutions. For those not used to or unhappy dealing with technical-looking manuals, checklists, and charts, the guide provides a very good introduction to gender and WASH programming.

Water Sanitation Hygiene (WASH): IASC Gender Marker Tip Sheet (2012), InterAgency Standing Committee (IASC), http://reliefweb.int/sites/reliefweb.int/files/resources/WASH2012TipSheet.pdf (last accessed 17 September 2019), 2 pp.

The IASC is a body co-ordinating humanitarian assistance between UN and non-UN organisations, and produces guidelines and tools for use in the humanitarian sector. The IASC Gender Marker is a tool used to assess how well gender is integrated into a project. 'Tip sheets' on gender equality in various aspects of humanitarian response, e.g. food security, health, and so on, form part of the tool, and this two-pager deals with gender equality in emergency WASH interventions. A checklist sets out key questions and considerations for needs assessments, and project activities and outcomes, and sample activities and indicators are provided to support project analysis and implementation.

'A framework for exploring gender equality outcomes from WASH programmes' (2013), Naomi Carrard, Joanne Crawford, Gabrielle Halcrow, Claire Rowland, and Juliet Willets, *Waterlines* 32(4): 315–33 (a pre-print version of this article is available at https://opus.lib.uts.edu.au/bitstream/10453/37894/1/Carrardetal2013_GenderOutcomesfromWASH_WaterlinesPreprint.pdf   (last accessed 17 September 2019)

Aiming to assist practitioners and researchers in planning, identifying, and documenting the gender outcomes of WASH programmes, the authors of this paper put forward a conceptual framework for classifying gender equality changes arising from WASH interventions. They argue that with gender outcomes that have been attributed to WASH initiatives encompassing those directly related to improved services as well as outcomes connected to relationships, power, and status, more work needs to be done in order to gain a better picture of the links between WASH and gender. Their framework is based on outcomes reported in WASH literature to date, empirical research in Fiji and Vanuatu, and insights from gender and development literature.

Infrastructure for All: Meeting the Needs of Both Men and Women in Development Projects – A Practical Guide for Engineers, Technicians and Project Managers

(2007) Brian Reed, Loughborough: Water, Engineering and Development Centre, University of Loughborough, http://wedc.lboro.ac.uk/resources/books/Infrastructure_for_All_-_Complete.pdf (last accessed 17 September 2019), 227 pp.

This is an excellent guide for those working on physical WASH infrastructure development, designed to help engineers and other technical staff understand the need for gender analysis in WASH projects. Seeking, as the book's foreword states, 'to give the "civil" aspects of their work equal weight with the "engineering" aspects', the book explains why an understanding of gender and other social relations will improve design, implementation, and use of engineers' technical interventions, and provides examples in the areas of water resources, water supply systems, and environmental sanitation, of infrastructure that has considered the needs of both women and men.

'Combining sanitation and women's participation in water supply: an example from Rajasthan' (2010) Kathleen O'Reilly, *Development in Practice* 20(1): 45–56

In this fascinating paper, the author describes a project where the well-intentioned, if illdefined, aims of women's participation and empowerment went awry. Because of a lack of attention to men's and women's different access to village and household spaces, a sanitation programme – in the form of the provision of household latrines – marketed as promoting women's empowerment and mobility, ended up (where the latrines were actually used, which was not always the case) creating reasons for women to remain in seclusion at home.

"Now we feel like respected adults": Positive change in gender roles and relations in a Timor Leste WASH program (2012) Di Kilsby, ACFID, WaterAid, IWDA, https://acfid.asn.au/sites/site.acfid/files/resource_document/Positive-change-in-genderroles-and-relations.pdf (last accessed 17 September 2019) 36 pp.

Published by the Australian Council for International Development, WaterAid and the International Women's Development Agency, this paper assesses the gendered outcomes of WaterAid's WASH programming in Timor Leste. Significant changes in both women's and men's lives were identified, and for women, positive changes in both their practical and strategic gender needs were found to have taken place. Some interesting differences were apparent in how women and men perceived and valued different kinds of change, with women, for example, valuing increased harmony in the home (deriving from reduced tensions around water provisioning), while this was barely noted by the men.

'Gender mainstreaming and water development projects: analyzing unexpected enviro-social impacts in Bolivia, India, and Lesotho' (2017) Maryann

R. Cairns, Cassandra L. Workman and Indrakshi Tandon, *Gender, Place and Culture* 24(3): 325–42

Using recent case studies from Bolivia, Lesotho, and India, the authors of this paper seek to address three questions: firstly, is mandatory inclusion of women in water governance and decision-making effective? Secondly, do water development projects provide equal benefits and burdens for women and men? And thirdly, in what ways are water projects affected by, and affecting, their gendered locations? Identifying major themes from all three contexts, the authors find that gender mainstreaming efforts are continuing to fall short in their aim of the equitable inclusion of women in their programming, and that specific geographic, environmental, and socio-cultural spaces are intimately related to how these equitability issues play out. Finally, the authors provide practical recommendations on how to address these issues.

Organisations

IRC, Bezuidenhoutseweg 2, 2594 AV, The Hague, The Netherlands, tel: +31 70 304 4000, email: via the website, website: www.ircwash.org

Founded in 1968 by the World Health Organization and the Dutch government as the International Reference Centre for Community Water Supply, IRC works as an international 'think-and-do tank', carrying out WASH programmes on the ground in 25 countries in Africa, Asia, and Latin America, and policy and advocacy work with NGOs, governments, and others, with an emphasis on providing long-term, sustainable solutions to the global crisis in WASH.

Rural Water and Sanitation Network (RWSN), c/o Skat Foundation, Vadianstrasse 42 St Gallen, CH-9000, Switzerland, email: ruralwater@skat.ch, website: www.rwsn.ch

RWSN is an international network of WASH professionals working in rural contexts. The network aims to share and develop knowledge and evidence, and raise standards in technical and professional competence, policy, and practice, with a particular focus on technologies and approaches that improve rural water supply.

Simavi, Naritaweg 135, 1043 BS Amsterdam, The Netherlands, tel: +31 88 313 15 00, email: info@simavi.nl, website: https://simavi.org

Working in the areas of WASH and sexual and reproductive health and rights (SRHR) in marginalised communities in Africa and Asia, this Dutch NGO focuses its programme work on behaviour change communication, menstrual hygiene management, maternal mortality audits, sustainable WASH services, and faecal sludge management.

WaterAid UK, 47–49 Durham Street, London SE11 5JD, UK, tel: +44 (0)20 7793 4594, email: supportercare@wateraid.org, website: www.wateraid.org/uk

Now part of a global confederation of WaterAids (with WaterAid Australia, WaterAid Sweden, and WaterAid America) the NGO WaterAid began in the UK in 1981. The organisation has become internationally recognised as a leader in the field, having developed much influential policy and practice on WASH. The website's Publications Library provides free access to many WaterAid resources, including research reports, training manuals, and policy briefings.

Water for People, 100 E. Tennessee Ave, Denver, CO 80209, USA, tel: +1 720 488 4590, email: info@waterforpeople.org, website: www.waterforpeople.org

This US-based NGO works to develop high-quality water and sanitation provision that is accessible to all, in nine countries – Honduras, Guatemala, Nicaragua, Bolivia, Peru, Malawi, Rwanda, Uganda, and India. Water for People's project model aims to provide 100 per cent WASH coverage in a specific, targeted region of a country, then replicate that in new regions, developing a scaleable strategy for providing sustainable services to communities that currently lack adequate WASH provision.

Water Supply and Sanitation Collaborative Council (WSSCC), 15, chemin LouisDunant, 1202 Geneva, Switzerland, tel: +41 (0)22 560 81 81, email: wsscc@wsscc.org, website: www.http://wsscc.org

WSSCC is hosted by the United Nations Office of Project Services, and is a global membership organisation made up of WASH professionals working through programmes and policy and advocacy development, to ensure sustainable WASH provision for all, with a focus on the poorest and most marginalised members of society in lowand middleincome countries in Africa and Asia. As well as providing a forum for collaboration and knowledge-sharing in the sector, WSSCC operates the Global Sanitation Fund, which is funded by donor governments, and has provided over US$112 million to WASH programmes in 13 developing countries since its inception in 2008.

Water, Engineering and Development Centre (WEDC), School of Civil and Building Engineering, The John Pickford Building, Loughborough University, Loughborough LE11 3TU, UK, tel: +44 (0)1509 222885, email: wedc@lboro.ac.uk, website: http://wedc.lboro.ac.uk

WEDC is an academic and research institute, with a global reputation in the field of WASH. It offers Masters and PhD-level teaching and research, with a focus on developing knowledge and capacity in water and sanitation for lowand middle-income countries. The annual WEDC Conference is a major international event for WASH-sector professionals, and serves as a learning event providing knowledge exchange and continued professional development for those working in the sector.

Oxfam GB is a development, relief, and campaigning organization that works with others to find lasting solutions to poverty and suffering around the world. Oxfam GB is a member of Oxfam International.

As part of its programme work, Oxfam undertakes research and documents its programme and humanitarian experience. This is disseminated through books, journals, policy papers, research reports, campaign reports, and other online products which are available for free download at: www.oxfam.org.uk/publications

www.oxfam.org.uk
Email: publish@oxfam.org.uk
Tel: +44 (0) 1865 473727

Oxfam House
John Smith Drive
Cowley
Oxford
OX4 2JY

The chapters in this book are available to download from the website: www.oxfam.org.uk/publications

www.ingramcontent.com/pod-product-compliance
Lightning Source LLC
Chambersburg PA
CBHW060324030426
42336CB00011B/1192